Hepatitis B Virus

Editor

TAREK I. HASSANEIN

CLINICS IN
LIVER DISEASE

www.liver.theclinics.com

Consulting Editor
NORMAN GITLIN

November 2016 • Volume 20 • Number 4

ELSEVIER

1600 John F. Kennedy Boulevard • Suite 1800 • Philadelphia, Pennsylvania, 19103-2899

http://www.theclinics.com

CLINICS IN LIVER DISEASE Volume 20, Number 4
November 2016 ISSN 1089-3261, ISBN-13: 978-0-323-47686-7

Editor: Kerry Holland
Developmental Editor: Meredith Clinton

Clinics in Liver Disease (ISSN 1089-3261) is published quarterly by Elsevier Inc., 360 Park Avenue South, New York, NY 10010-1710. Months of issue are February, May, August, and November. Business and Editorial Offices: 1600 John F. Kennedy Blvd., Ste. 1800, Philadelphia, PA 19103-2899. Customer Service Office: 3251 Riverport Lane, Maryland Heights, MO 63043. Periodicals postage paid at New York, NY and additional mailing offices. Subscription prices are $275.00 per year (U.S. individuals), $100.00 per year (U.S. student/resident), $453.00 per year (U.S. institutions), $395.00 per year (international individuals), $200.00 per year (international student/resident), $562.00 per year (international instituitions), $340.00 per year (Canadian individuals), $200.00 per year (Canadian student/resident), and $562.00 per year (Canadian institutions). Foreign air speed delivery is included in all *Clinics* subscription prices. All prices are subject to change without notice. **POSTMASTER:** Send address changes to *Clinics in Liver Disease*, Elsevier Health Sciences Division, Subscription Customer Service, 3251 Riverport Lane, Maryland Heights, MO 63043. **Customer Service: Telephone: 1-800-654-2452 (U.S. and Canada); 314-447-8871 (outside U.S. and Canada). Fax: 314-447-8029. E-mail: journalscustomer service-usa@elsevier.com (for print support); journalsonlinesupport-usa@elsevier.com (for online support).**

Reprints. For copies of 100 or more of articles in this publication, please contact the Commercial Reprints Department, Elsevier Inc., 360 Park Avenue South, New York, NY 10010-1710. Tel.: 212-633-3874; Fax: 212-633-3820; E-mail: reprints@elsevier.com.

Clinics in Liver Disease is covered in *MEDLINE/PubMed (Index Medicus)*, Science Citation Index Expanded, Journal Citation Reports/Science Edition, and Current Contents/Clinical Medicine.

Contributors

CONSULTING EDITOR

NORMAN GITLIN, MD, FRCP (LONDON), FRCPE (EDINBURGH), FAASLD, FACP, FACG
Formerly, Professor of Medicine, Chief of Hepatology, Emory University; Currently, Consultant, Atlanta Gastroenterology Associates, Atlanta, Georgia

EDITOR

TAREK I. HASSANEIN, MD, FACP, FACG, AGAF, FAASLD
Professor of Medicine, University of California San Diego School of Medicine; Director, Southern California Liver Centers, San Diego, California; Medical Director, Southern California Research Center, Coronado, California

AUTHORS

LEDA BASSIT, PhD
Laboratory of Biochemical Pharmacology, Department of Pediatrics, Center for AIDS Research, Emory University School of Medicine, Atlanta, Georgia

BERTRAM BENGSCH, MD, PhD
Department of Microbiology, Institute for Immunology, Perelman School of Medicine, University of Pennsylvania, Philadelphia, Pennsylvania

JENNIFER BERUMEN, MD
Assistant Professor of Surgery, Division of Transplantation and Hepatobiliary Surgery, University of California San Diego, La Jolla, California

SEBASTIEN BOUCLE, PhD
Laboratory of Biochemical Pharmacology, Department of Pediatrics, Center for AIDS Research, Emory University School of Medicine, Atlanta, Georgia

KYONG-MI CHANG, MD
Associate Chief of Staff for Research, Medical Research; Associate Dean for Research, Philadelphia Corporal Michael J. Crescenz VA Medical Center (CMC VAMC); Associate Professor of Medicine, Gastroenterology Division, Perelman School of Medicine, University of Pennsylvania, Philadelphia, Pennsylvania

PING-YU CHEN, MD
Department of Medicine, University of California Los Angeles, Los Angeles, California

PHILIPPA J. EASTERBROOK, MD, MPH
Senior Scientist, HIV/AIDS Department, World Health Organization, Geneva, Switzerland

MARYAM EHTESHAMI, PhD
Laboratory of Biochemical Pharmacology, Department of Pediatrics, Center for AIDS Research, Emory University School of Medicine, Atlanta, Georgia

TAREK I. HASSANEIN, MD, FACP, FACG, AGAF, FAASLD
Professor of Medicine, University of California San Diego School of Medicine; Director, Southern California Liver Centers, San Diego, California; Medical Director, Southern California Research Center, Coronado, California

ALAN W. HEMMING, MD, MSc, FRCSC, FACS
Professor and Chief, Division of Transplantation and Hepatobiliary Surgery, University of California San Diego, La Jolla, California

MONICA A. KONERMAN, MD, MSc
Division of Gastroenterology, Department of Internal Medicine, University of Michigan Health System, Ann Arbor, Michigan

RYAN M. KWOK, MD
Gastroenterology/Transplant Hepatology; Associate Program Director, Gastroenterology Fellowship Program, Walter Reed National Military Medical Center; Assistant Professor of Medicine, Uniformed Services University, Bethesda, Maryland

ANNA S. LOK, MD
Division of Gastroenterology, Department of Internal Medicine, University of Michigan Health System, Ann Arbor, Michigan

BRENDON K. LUVISA, BA
Southern California Research Center, Coronado, California

BRIAN J. McMAHON, MD
Affiliate Professor of WWAMI School of Medical Education, University of Alaska, Anchorage, Alaska

KRISTIN MEKEEL, MD
Professor of Surgery, Division of Transplantation and Hepatobiliary Surgery, University of California San Diego, La Jolla, California

NOELE P. NELSON, MD, PhD, MPH
Medical Epidemiologist, Centers for Disease Control and Prevention, Atlanta, Georgia

DON C. ROCKEY, MD
Department of Internal Medicine; Professor and Chairman, Department of Medicine, The Medical University of South Carolina, Charleston, South Carolina

CLARA E. SAAB, BA
Department of Surgery, University of California Los Angeles, Los Angeles, California

SAMMY SAAB, MD, MPH, AGAF, FAASLD, FACG
Departments of Surgery and Medicine, University of California Los Angeles, Los Angeles, California

RAYMOND F. SCHINAZI, PhD, DSc
Laboratory of Biochemical Pharmacology, Department of Pediatrics, Center for AIDS Research, Emory University School of Medicine, Atlanta, Georgia

MYRON J. TONG, MD, PhD
Department of Surgery, University of California Los Angeles, Los Angeles, California; Huntington Medical Research Institutes, Pasadena, California

TRAM T. TRAN, MD
Medical Director Liver Transplant; Professor of Medicine; Director, Gastroenterology Fellowship Program, Cedars Sinai Medical Center, Geffen School of Medicine at University of California Los Angeles, Los Angeles, California

Contents

Integration of hepatitis B vaccination into national immunization programs has resulted in substantial reductions of hepatitis B virus (HBV) transmission in previously high endemic countries. The key strategy for control of the HBV epidemic is birth dose and infant vaccination. Additional measures include use of hepatitis B immunoglobulin (HBIG) and diagnosis of mothers at high risk of transmitting HBV and use of antiviral agents during pregnancy to decrease maternal DNA concentrations to undetectable concentrations. Despite the substantial decrease in HBV cases since vaccination introduction, implementation of birth dose vaccination in low-income and middle-income countries and vaccination of high-risk adults remain challenging.

Hepatitis B virus (HBV) infection is a major global health challenge. HBV can cause significant morbidity and mortality by establishing acute and chronic hepatitis. Approximately 250 million people worldwide are chronically infected, and more than 2 billion people have been exposed to HBV. Since the discovery of HBV, the advances in our understanding of HBV virology and immunology have translated into effective vaccines and therapies for HBV infection. Although current therapies successfully suppress viral replication but rarely succeed in viral eradication, recent discoveries in HBV virology and immunology provide exciting rationales for novel treatment strategies aiming at HBV cure.

Chronic hepatitis B virus (HBV) infection has a significant public health impact. There are currently 7 approved therapies for chronic HBV, including standard and pegylated interferon (IFN)-α, and 5 nucleos(t)ide analogs (NUCs). IFN offers benefits over NUCs, including a finite duration of therapy and a higher rate of clearance of hepatitis B e antigen and surface antigen. These benefits need to be weighed against the potential adverse effects of IFN therapy. Some patients should not receive IFN because of advanced liver disease or comorbidities. This article reviews the mechanisms of action, efficacy, and clinical use of IFN therapy for HBV infection.

with the development of HCC in hepatitis B, along with advances in the diagnosis, imaging, and management of HCC.

Liver transplant (LT) is now an established indication for patients with chronic hepatitis B, mainly because of the development and use of hepatitis B immunoglobulin (HBIG) and oral antivirals for prophylaxis. The combination of low-dose HBIG and antivirals has been considered the standard prophylaxis regimen to prevent post-LT recurrence of hepatitis B. The important remaining issues are related to the long-term cost of HBIG and the risk of escape hepatitis B virus (HBV) mutants. Strategies for prevention of HBV after LT are constantly improving. With the availability of new nucleoside/nucleotide analogues, new post-LT strategies should also emerge.

Hepatitis B virus (HBV) causes significant morbidity and mortality worldwide. The majority of chronically infected individuals do not achieve a functional and complete cure. Treated persons who achieve a long-term sustained virologic response (undetectable HBV DNA), are still at high risk of developing morbidity and mortality from liver complications. This review focuses on novel, mechanistically diverse anti-HBV therapeutic strategies currently in development or in clinical evaluation, and highlights new combination strategies that may contribute to full elimination of HBV DNA and covalently closed circular DNA from the infected liver, leading to a complete cure of chronic hepatitis B.

CLINICS IN LIVER DISEASE

THE CLINICS ARE AVAILABLE ONLINE!
Access your subscription at:
www.theclinics.com

Preface

Hepatitis B Virus: The Past, The Present, and The Future

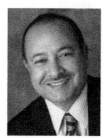

Tarek I. Hassanein, MD, FACP, FACG, AGAF, FAASLD
Editor

Hepatitis B virus (HBV) is a unique DNA virus with worldwide distribution infecting millions of individuals and causing progressive liver disease and cancer in many patients. Despite the availability of effective vaccines, challenges still persist in different parts of the world in implementing global vaccination efforts. Drs Nelson, Easterbrook, and McMahon discuss the epidemiology of HBV and the current situation of HBV vaccination. As our understanding of the virus replication and interaction with the human immune system improves, we can tailor viral inhibition and ameliorate viral effects on the liver and the patient as a whole. Drs Bengsch and Chang take us on a journey exploring the HBV virology and its interactions with the human immune system. With the recent advances in oral antivirals, new data continue to show the beneficial effect of immune modulators such as interferons in subgroups of patients with active HBV infection. Drs Konerman and Lok briefly review the current indications for the use of interferons in an era of highly active hepatitis B antivirals. The goal of curing HBV is still unreachable, but the current therapies effectively impact the viral replications and improve hepatic inflammation and liver fibrosis. Dr Rockey covers the dynamic processes of fibrogenesis and the effects of antivirals on liver injury and fibrosis. Delay in the diagnosis and the use of antivirals may result in patient disease progression causing liver decompensation. Drs Luvisa and Hassanein cover the approach of managing patients with liver decompensation and those who need liver transplantation. Patients with chronic HBV infection continue to have a risk for hepatocellular carcinoma (HCC) and non-HCC cancers. Drs Kwok and Tran address the issue of non-HCC cancer in patients chronically infected with HBV. The role of surgery in patients with HCC is detailed by Drs Hemming, Berumen, and Mekeel. A subset of patients who continue to suffer the ravages of HBV infection ultimately benefit from liver transplantation. Managing patients who receive a liver transplant is costly and sometimes difficult. Drs S. Saab, Chen, C. Saab, and Tong discuss the different approaches for managing HBV after liver transplantation. Although the current Hepatitis B antiviral therapies are readily

Clin Liver Dis 20 (2016) ix–x
http://dx.doi.org/10.1016/j.cld.2016.08.014
1089-3261/16/© 2016 Published by Elsevier Inc.

liver.theclinics.com

available and highly effective in suppressing viral replication and disease progression in the great majority of patients, achieving cure is still far away. Drs Boucle, Bassit, Ehteshami, and Schinazi end the issue with a glimpse of the new approaches to achieve the ultimate goal of cure. This issue of the *Clinics of Liver Disease* gathered a distinguished faculty discussing the most recent data surrounding the past, present, and future of HBV. Many thanks to the faculty for their participation, and the editorial team for their exhaustive efforts in putting this issue together.

Tarek I. Hassanein, MD, FACP, FACG, AGAF, FAASLD
University of California
San Diego School of Medicine
San Diego, CA, USA

Southern California Liver Centers
San Diego, CA, USA

Southern California Research Center
PO Box 181770
Coronado, CA 92178-1770, USA

E-mail address:
thassanein@livercenters.com

Epidemiology of Hepatitis B Virus Infection and Impact of Vaccination on Disease

Noele P. Nelson, MD, PhD, MPH[a],*, Philippa J. Easterbrook, MD, MPH[b],
Brian J. McMahon, MD[c]

KEYWORDS

- Hepatitis B virus • Hepatitis B vaccine • Birth dose • Perinatal transmission
- Vaccine impact

KEY POINTS

- The Global Advisory Group of the Expanded Programme on Immunization recommendations to integrate hepatitis B vaccination into national immunization programs have resulted in substantial reductions of hepatitis B virus (HBV) transmission in previously high endemic countries.
- A 68% decrease in HBV infection prevalence among US children, regardless of country of origin, was observed within 10 years of initiation of universal hepatitis B vaccination.
- The key strategy for control of the HBV epidemic is universal infant vaccination with administration of birth dose and 3 doses of hepatitis B vaccine in the first year of life. Additional measures include use of hepatitis B immunoglobulin (HBIG) and together with diagnosis of mothers at high risk of transmitting HBV with use of antiviral agents in the late first or early second trimester to decrease maternal DNA concentrations to undetectable concentrations.
- Despite the substantial decrease in HBV cases since vaccination introduction, implementation of birth dose vaccination in low-income and middle-income countries and vaccination of high-risk adults remain challenging.

INTRODUCTION
Global Hepatitis B Virus Burden

Hepatitis B virus (HBV) infection is a global public health problem.[1,2] Worldwide estimates suggest that more than 2 billion people have been infected with HBV, and that 248 million of these people are chronically infected (defined as hepatitis B surface

Disclosure: The authors have nothing to disclose.
[a] Clinical Interventions Team, National Center for HIV/AIDS, Viral Hepatitis, STD, and TB Prevention, Centers for Disease Control and Prevention, 1600 Clifton Road, MS-G37, Atlanta, GA 30329-4018, USA; [b] Global Hepatitis Programme, HIV Department, World Health Organization, 20 Via Appia, Geneva 1211, Switzerland; [c] Liver Disease and Hepatitis Program, Alaska Native Medical Center, Alaska Native Tribal Health Consortium, 4315 Diplomacy Drive, Anchorage, AK 99508, USA
* Corresponding author.
E-mail address: nnelson@cdc.gov

antigen [HBsAg] positivity).[3] About 15% to 25% of persons with chronic HBV infection die from cirrhosis or liver cancer.[3] The Global Burden of Disease study estimated that there were 686,000 deaths caused by hepatitis B in 2013 and a 5.9 per 100,000 age-standardized death rate globally,[4] of which 300,000 deaths were attributed to liver cancer and 317,400 deaths to cirrhosis of the liver secondary to hepatitis B.[4] This rate represents a substantial global burden, with wide global geographic variation. Hepatitis B prevalence (HBsAg) is highest in the sub-Saharan African and western Pacific regions, considered high-intermediate to high endemicity countries (5% to ≥8% prevalence), and prevalence estimates exceed 15% in several countries. Low-intermediate regions (2%–4.99%) include the eastern Mediterranean and European regions. The Americas and Western Europe regions are considered low endemicity, with HBsAg prevalence generally less than 2%.[3,5] There has been an overall decrease in HBsAg prevalence over time in most countries, but with notable increases in African and eastern European countries.[3]

United States Hepatitis B Virus Burden

In the United States, estimates of chronic hepatitis B infection range from 700,000 to more than 2 million people.[6–9] Estimating the number of chronically infected persons globally and in the United States is challenging because the disease is asymptomatic in most infected persons, leading to underdiagnosis, and passive surveillance often results in under reporting.[7,9] Despite declines in chronic hepatitis B cases among children and adolescents, due to increasing immunity following universal vaccine recommendations, the number of chronically infected adults in the United States has been increasing as a result of immigration of infected persons from highly endemic countries.[10,11] As many as 70% of HBV infections in the United States are estimated to be among foreign-born persons.[12] Yearly, 40,000 to 45,000 people from HBV-endemic countries where the prevalence of chronic HBV infection is >2%, enter the United States legally[11]; an estimated 3.9 million foreign-born persons from eastern Asia and sub-Saharan Africa currently reside in the United States.[13]

The prevalence of HBV infection is analyzed each year by the National Health and Examination Survey (NHANES), a survey representative of the US noninstitutionalized household population.[6,14] Recent NHANES data from 2011 to 2012 indicate that there are approximately 850,000 Americans living with chronic HBV infection in the United States.[9] Oversampling of non-Hispanic Asians, who represent about 5% of the US population, indicate that non-Hispanic Asians account for almost 50% (400,000) of all chronic HBV infections in the United States.[12,15]

In the United States, rates of acute infection have remained about 1.0 per 100,000 population since 2009, and have been reported from more nonurban than urban regions.[16] African American adults have the highest rate of acute HBV infection in the United States.[15] Recently (2006–2013) an increase in incident cases of acute HBV infection in Kentucky, Tennessee, and West Virginia has occurred among non-Hispanic white people aged 30 to 39 years, who reported injection-drug use as a common risk factor.[17]

TRANSMISSION OF HEPATITIS B VIRUS

There are 2 major modes of transmission of HBV that occur in the world. Perinatal transmission, occurring at birth from infected mothers to their newborns, accounts for the majority of HBV transmission worldwide. Horizontal transmission can occur through open cuts and scratches; transfusion of blood products; breaks in good practices to prevent blood-borne infections in the health care setting; sexual transmission and risky behavior, including injecting-drug use or tattooing, body piercing, and scar-ification procedures without the use of sterilized equipment and needles.

The risk of developing chronic HBV infection among susceptible persons decreases with age at infection and thus depends on the mode of transmission. Up to 90% of perinatal infections become chronically infected; approximately 20% to 60% of children aged 1 to 5 years become chronically infected, and 5% to 10% of older children and adults.[18–21]

Perinatal Transmission

Hepatitis B "e" antigen (HBeAg) is a serologic marker for high viral levels of HBV DNA. Perinatal transmission occurs almost universally in mothers who are positive for but also can occur in mothers who have very high levels of HBV DNA, > 200,000 IU/ml in their blood. The risk of an unvaccinated infant acquiring HBV at birth is up to 100% in an infant born to an HBeAg-positive mother. The classic study by Palmer Beasley in Taiwan in the 1970's, before vaccine was available, demon-strated that among women who were HBeAg-positive, 85% of their infants became chronically infected as compared to 32% among HBeAg negative women.[22] An estimated 90% risk of developing chronic HBV exists among infants infected perinatally.

Prevention of Perinatal Transmission

The most impactful strategy for reducing mother to newborn transmission of HBV is incorporating the birth dose into the hepatitis B vaccine schedule. A birth dose fol-lowed by 2 more doses of hepatitis B vaccine can reduce the prevalence of chronic HBV in the infant by approximately 90% in infants of HBeAg-positive mothers and almost all HBeAg-negative mothers. This birth dose is especially important in areas of the world where a significant proportion of HBsAg-positive mothers are also pos-itive for HBeAg, such as in China, south east Asia, and the Pacific Islands. In these areas, if the birth dose is not given, the effectiveness of hepatitis B vaccine could be reduced to as low as only 50% to 75%.[23] In regions such as sub-Saharan Africa and Russia where less than 25% of HBsAg-positive pregnant women are also HBeAg positive,[24] the impact of missing the birth dose is not as severe but is still significant. Including a dose of HBIG at birth to infants born to HBsAg-positive mothers can further reduce the risk of transmission to less than 5%. Beasley and his colleagues showed in a randomized-controlled trial, that with administration of the birth dose plus HBIG to infants born to HBsAg/HBeAg-positive mothers only 6% of those infants became HBsAg-positive verses 88% of infants who received placebo.[25]

Horizontal Transmission

Horizontal transmission of HBV, if it occurs in young children, has a high risk of leading to chronic HBV. Three prospective studies conducted before the availability of hepatitis B vaccine have shown this.[26–28] A study of 1280 persons who were seronegative for HBV markers conducted in Alaskan villages in the 1970s found that, of 189 persons who acquired HBV during a 4-year period, 29% of those less than the age of 5 years developed chronic HBV versus 16% of those between 5 and 10 years and 8% of those more than 30 years of age.[26] In a study from Taiwan following children born without HBV infection who acquired HBV before 5 years of age, 23% developed chronic HBV.[27] A third study from Senegal found that 50% of children infected horizontally before the age of 2 years became chronically infected.[28] In the Senegal study the rate of chronic HBV decreased from 68% at 1 year to 6.3% after 4 years of age. Furthermore, for those infected at less than 6 months of age, the rate of chronic HBV was 82%, and for those infected between 6 months and 1 year it was 54%. Inclusion of the birth dose and subsequent doses not only prevents perinatal transmission but also reduces acquisition of infection in the first few months of life when there is the greatest risk of developing chronic infection via horizontal transmission.

In young children and some adults, horizontal transmission likely occurs because of the presence of infectious HBV on environmental surfaces. In a study from Alaska 40 years ago, before HBV DNA testing was available, HBsAg was found by environmental sampling on school lunch room table tops; on walls, toys, and baby bottles in homes where HBsAg-positive persons were living; and filtered from impetigo sores.[29] Furthermore, when HBV was left at room temperature, after at least 7 days viral replication was found to occur.[30] Virus may be shed via open cuts, scratches, and sores from persons with chronic HBV onto environmental surfaces and then can infect other persons with open lesions through their contact with the contaminated surfaces. Horizontal transmission also occurs via unsterile injections from health care encounters or injection-drug use and tattooing as well as scarification practices, sexual transmission, and via high-risk health care environments, including renal dialysis units and emergency rooms.[31]

Among young adults in the United States, injection-drug use is an increasing cause of horizontal hepatitis B transmission in some areas. A 114% increase in acute HBV infection from 2006 to 2013 was found in Kentucky, Tennessee, and West Virginia.[17] The increase occurred primarily among white people aged 30 to 39 years who reported the use of injection-drugs. Outbreaks in health care settings is a further cause of horizontal transmission. From 2008 to 2014, 23 acute hepatitis B outbreaks occurred related to health care.[32] These outbreaks were associated with 175 cases and more than 10,700 persons were notified for screening. Of these outbreaks, 17 outbreaks occurred in long-term care facilities, and most were associated with infection-control lapses during assisted monitoring of blood glucose levels.[32]

Prevention of horizontal transmission requires education, appropriate infection-control practices, and vaccination of hepatitis B household contacts and other persons at high risk of hepatitis B.

STRATEGIES FOR CONTROL AND PREVENTION OF HEPATITIS B INFECTION

This article discusses the good practice principals that can effectively halt transmission of HBV. It uses as examples global and US programs in HBV vaccination (eg, Alaska) to demonstrate how effective infant vaccination strategies can accomplish this goal, starting with the first dose of hepatitis B vaccine administered immediately after birth followed by full vaccination during infancy and the use of catch-up vaccination programs for children. In addition, it highlights how programs targeting adults at the highest risk of HBV infection can prevent acute icteric HBV infection and transmission in this age group.

Global Vaccine Policy

In 1991, the Global Advisory Group of the Expanded Programme on Immunization (EPI) recommended integration of hepatitis B vaccination into national immunization programs by 1995 in countries with an HBV carrier prevalence of 8% or higher, and by 1997 in countries with a lower prevalence.[2] By the end of 2014, hepatitis B vaccine had been introduced nationwide in 184 countries.[1,2]

World Health Organization Recommendations and Strategy on Vaccination for Control of Hepatitis B

There are 5 key World Health Organization (WHO) strategic areas for hepatitis B prevention through vaccination summarised in a WHO policy document from the Western Pacific region.[33]

Vaccination of infants

The WHO recommends the use of monovalent HBV vaccination within 24 hours of birth, followed by completion of the HBV vaccine series within 6 to 12 months as the most cost-effective strategy for the prevention and control of hepatitis B.[33,34] This strategy provides the earliest possible protection to future birth cohorts and reduces the pool of chronic carriers in the population. Timely vaccination of newborn infants can prevent perinatal HBV transmission. **Table 1** shows a typical schedule of hepatitis B and pentavalent vaccination in the western Pacific region. Strengthening of routine immunization services to achieve and sustain high coverage with 3 doses of hepatitis B vaccine by 1 year of age is the most important strategy for hepatitis B control. Mathematical modeling suggests that very high vaccine coverage rates ($\geq$ 90%) are needed to interrupt transmission and prevent deaths, with the goal to protect the entire birth cohort and achieve health equity.[35]

Delivery of a timely birth dose also provides an opportunity to link immunization delivery systems with maternal health programs, and to ensure that HBV vaccine is included in the essential care package for newborn infants, and to harmonize training and programmatic issues, including where, when, and by whom the birth dose is given.

Hepatitis B immune globulin (HBIG) Where resources allow, HBIG may be given in addition to the vaccine to children born to HBsAg-positive mothers. However, the option for HBIG is conditional on the existence of a comprehensive antenatal screening

Table 1
Typical schedule of hepatitis B (HepB) and pentavalent (diphtheria-tetanus-pertussis [DTP], Haemophilus influenzae B [Hib], HepB) vaccination in the Western Pacific Region

Age[a]	Vaccine
At birth (within 24 h)	HepB monovalent
6 wk	DTP-HepB-Hib1
10 wk	DTP-HepB-Hib2
14 wk	DTP-HepB-Hib3

Although 3 doses are sufficient to induce immunity, for programmatic reasons most countries in the region use a combination vaccine, resulting in a 4-dose schedule.

[a] Ages given are recommended as the earliest possible, but they are flexible. Immunization programs should emphasize vaccination at birth and completing the hepatitis B series by 6 months of age.

Data from Hepatitis B control through immunization: a reference guide. Available at: http://www.who.int/immunization/sage/meetings/2015/october/8_WPRO_Hepatitis_B_Prevention_Through_Immunization_Regional_Reference_Guide.pdf.

program for hepatitis B infection, and is of limited value in settings with poor antenatal coverage.[33]

Catch-up vaccination The WHO also recommends catch-up vaccination for older children who missed immunization as infants as a secondary strategy after routine vaccination reaches target levels. This strategy depends on whether a country has additional financial and human resources for enhanced hepatitis B control, and should be based on careful epidemiologic and economic analysis.

Vaccination of priority adult population groups may be prioritized after infant immunization

Priority or high-risk population groups include health care workers, contacts of HBsAg-positive persons, men who have sex with men, sex workers, people who inject drugs, frequent recipients of blood/plasma transfusions, and any other population groups coming in regular contact with blood and blood products. Incidence of acute HBV is highest among adolescents and adults, although the risk of developing chronic HBV is low compared with infants and children. Vaccination programs targeting high-risk adults can be difficult to implement because of challenges in identifying and vaccinating persons engaged in high-risk activity before they become infected. Universal vaccination of health care workers is an effective strategy to protect high-risk adult groups from HBV infection.[36]

Vaccine supply and quality

Key goals are elimination of vaccine stock-outs at the national and district levels through improved training in vaccine management, prevention of vaccine freezing through improved training in temperature monitoring, and promotion of the use of controlled temperature chain for hepatitis B birth dose delivery.[33]

Advocacy and social mobilization

The primary goal is to increase awareness among decision makers, health care workers, and caretakers of the risks and consequences of HBV infection and the need for hepatitis B vaccination through community and civil society engagement, use of media outlets, education materials, and mass awareness campaigns such as World Hepatitis Day and World immunization week.[33]

Measurement of program performance and impact

Because frequent serologic surveys are not feasible, vaccine coverage rates serve as an interim proxy for program performance, and can help identify areas of poor performance where increased resources and efforts should be focused. Although routinely collected administrative data may be used for regular monitoring, it is useful to supplement this with periodic vaccination coverage surveys to identify any major problems. Such surveys usually target children aged 12 to 33 months to allow estimation of vaccine coverage for the most recent birth cohort. In order to assess the status of the impact of the vaccination program, seroprevalence surveys are essential. There is no set schedule for conducting these surveys and they should be undertaken when it is programmatically important to do so.[33]

VACCINATION OF INFANTS AND ADMINISTRATION OF HEPATITIS B IMMUNE GLOBULIN
United States Vaccine Policy

In the United States in 1991, the Advisory Committee on Immunization Practices (ACIP) published a comprehensive strategy for eliminating transmission in the United

States through universal childhood. The strategy included recommendations for the prevention of perinatal HBV infection, universal vaccination of infants born to HBsAg-negative mothers, vaccination of adolescents, and vaccination of selected high-risk groups.[37] The recommendations have been revised and expanded since 1991.

United States Universal Infant and Childhood and Adult Vaccination Policy

The 2005 ACIP recommendations[38] state that infants born to mothers who are HBsAg-positive should receive hepatitis B vaccine and HBIG within the first 12 hours of birth. Infants born to mothers whose HBsAg status is unknown should receive hepatitis B vaccine in the first 12 hours after birth. The mother should have blood drawn as soon as possible to determine her HBsAg status; if she is HBsAg-positive, the infant should receive HBIG as soon as possible (no later than age 1 week). Full-term infants who are medically stable and weigh more than 2000 g born to HBsAg-negative mothers should receive single-antigen hepatitis B vaccine before hospital discharge. Preterm infants weighing less than 2000 g born to HBsAg-negative mothers should receive the first dose of vaccine 1 month after birth or at hospital discharge.[38]

After the birth dose, all infants should complete the hepatitis B vaccine series with either single-antigen vaccine or combination vaccine, according to a recommended vaccination schedule[38] (**Box 1**). Postvaccination serologic testing consisting of HBsAg and anti-HBs should be ordered at age 9 to 12 months (or 1–2 months after the final dose of the vaccine series, if delayed) for infants born to HBsAg-positive mothers only,[39] to enable prompt identification and revaccination of nonresponders who were exposed at birth.

Catch-up Vaccination

All unvaccinated children and adolescents aged less than 19 years old should receive the hepatitis B vaccine series according to the hepatitis B catch-up schedule.[40]

Adult Vaccination

High-risk adults should also receive the 3 doses of hepatitis B vaccine[41] (**Box 2**). High-risk adults include persons at risk for infection by sexual exposure, and persons at risk for infection by percutaneous or mucosal exposure to blood and other infectious fluids. Persons at risk of sexual exposure include sex partners of HBsAg-positive persons; sexually active persons who are not in a long-term, mutually monogamous relationship; persons seeking evaluation or treatment of a sexually transmitted disease; and men who have sex with men. Persons at risk for percutaneous exposure include current or recent injection-drug users; household contacts of HBsAg-positive persons; residents and staff of facilities for developmentally disabled persons; health care and public safety workers with reasonably anticipated risk for exposure to blood or blood-contaminated body fluids; persons with end-stage renal disease, including predialysis, hemodialysis, peritoneal dialysis, and home dialysis patients. Others who should receive this vaccine include international travelers to regions with high or intermediate levels (HBsAg prevalence of $\geq 2\%$) of endemic HBV infection, persons with chronic liver disease, persons with human immunodeficiency virus (HIV) infection, and all other persons seeking protection from HBV infection (**Box 3**).[41]

Alaska Vaccination Program

In the 1970s epidemiologic studies found that HBV infection was endemic in western Alaska. Rates of acute icteric HBV infection were more than 200 per 100,000 and the prevalence of chronic HBV was 6% to 8%.[42] Furthermore, the incidence of hepatocellular carcinoma (HCC) was the highest in the United States at the time and was especially high in children and young adults.[43] Five different HBV genotypes were found in Alaska and, because of that, transmission was predominantly perinatal in northwest Alaska, where genotype C predominated, similar to what is observed in China and southeast Asia, but there was horizontal child to child transmission in southwest Alaska, similar to the predominant mode of transmission in Africa.[26,44] Studies from Alaska found that persons infected with genotype C on average cleared HBeAg after reaching their mid-40's and thus most were positive throughout most of their childbearing years. In contrast most of those infected with genotypes A, B6, D and F cleared HBeAg in the teens and early 20's early in their childbearing years.[44] The approach to interrupting transmission therefore had to address both the perinatal and horizontal routes. To accomplish this, a combination of vaccination starting at birth and 2 further doses, coupled with a rapid catch-up program was aimed at children as well as adults. The rationale for including adults was based on studies that showed that although children were passing the infection through open cuts and scratches, a large component of transmission in adults was sexual.[26,31]

The program began in 1980 with screening of pregnant women for HBsAg in the 2 largest hospitals serving Alaska Native (AN) persons in the state and administering HBIG at birth, 1 month, and 3 months to infants born of HBsAg-positive mothers. In 1981 and 1982, a trial with plasma-derived vaccine (Heptavax) was conducted in 16 villages in western Alaska in adults and children more than 6 months of ages and showed that this vaccine was highly efficacious in preventing transmission.[45] In 1984, funding was obtained to start a statewide comprehensive program designed to completely eradicate transmission of HBV in the AN population.

Over the next 4 years, 53,000 AN persons were tested for HBV serologic markers, which represented two-thirds of the statewide AN population and 90% of children and adults living in western Alaska; 40,000 serologically negative persons were vaccinated.[46,47] In addition, in all hospitals, screening of pregnant women with HBsAg was initiated and infants of HBsAg-positive mothers received both HBIG and 3 doses of hepatitis B vaccination starting at birth, plus universal vaccination was initiated for all infants, starting with a birth dose. Since the mid-1990s, universal hepatitis B vaccination has been given to all newborns in Alaska, regardless of race or ethnicity, starting at birth, and there has been a catch-up program for all children through age 19 years consistent with the ACIP recommendations.

IMPACT OF VACCINATION GLOBALLY AND IN THE UNITED STATES
Impact and Current Status of Implementation of World Health Organization Recommendations

The 1991 EPI recommendations for universal hepatitis B vaccine at birth and other hepatitis B vaccination strategies have resulted in substantial reductions of HBV transmission in previously high endemic countries.[2] In 2014, global coverage with 3 doses of hepatitis B vaccine is estimated at 82% (compared to 1% in 1990) and is as high as 92% in the Western Pacific.[1] For example, the national Taiwan vaccine program, which started in 1984, has been 78% to 87% effective in reducing HBsAg seroprevalence in children.[48] China has also made remarkable progress in increasing immunization coverage of hepatitis B vaccine. From 2005 to 2009, demonstration projects

---

Box 1
Hepatitis B (HepB) vaccine in the United States (minimum age: birth)

Routine vaccination:

At birth:
- Administer monovalent HepB vaccine to all newborns before hospital discharge.
- For infants born to HBsAg-positive mothers, administer HepB vaccine and 0.5 mL of HBIG within 12 hours of birth. These infants should be tested for HBsAg and anti-HBs at age 9 to 12 months (preferably at the next well-child visit) or 1 to 2 months after completion of the HepB series if the series was delayed; see http://www.cdc.gov/mmwr/preview/mmwrhtml/mm6439a6.htm.
- If mother's HBsAg status is unknown, within 12 hours of birth administer HepB vaccine regardless of birth weight.
- For infants weighing less than 2000 g, administer HBIG in addition to HepB vaccine within 12 hours of birth. Determine the mother's HBsAg status as soon as possible and, if the mother is HBsAg-positive, also administer HBIG for infants weighing 2000 g or more as soon as possible, but no later than age 7 days.

Doses following the birth dose:

- The second dose should be administered at age 1 or 2 months. Monovalent HepB vaccine should be used for doses administered before age 6 weeks.

- Infants who did not receive a birth dose should receive 3 doses of a HepB-containing vaccine on a schedule of 0, 1 to 2 months, and 6 months starting as soon as feasible.

- Administer the second dose 1 to 2 months after the first dose (minimum interval of 4 weeks), administer the third dose at least 8 weeks after the second dose and at least 16 weeks after the first dose. The final (third or fourth) dose in the HepB vaccine series should be administered no earlier than age 24 weeks.

- Administration of a total of 4 doses of HepB vaccine is permitted when a combination vaccine containing HepB is administered after the birth dose.

Catch-up vaccination:

- Unvaccinated persons should complete a 3-dose series.

- A 2-dose series (doses separated by at least 4 months) of adult formulation Recombivax HB® is licensed for use in children aged 11 through 15 years.

Data from http://www.cdc.gov/vaccines/schedules/hcp/child-adolescent.html. Accessed August 15, 2016.

---

focused on promoting hospital delivery, strengthening collaboration between the EPI and the maternal and child health program, and developing strategies for both hospital and home births.[49]

By the end of 2014, hepatitis B vaccine had been introduced nationwide in 184 countries. **Fig. 1** shows the geographic variation in coverage of the third dose of HBV vaccine in 2014. **Fig. 2** shows the temporal trends in vaccination coverage for both the third dose and birth dose in the western Pacific region, and the marked increases in coverage that occurred in 2000 and 2004 respectively. A birth dose for hepatitis B vaccine was introduced in 96 countries by 2014, and global coverage was estimated at 38%, reaching 80% in the western Pacific, but only 10% in the African region.[50] Data from 2012 also show that only 52% of countries recommend giving the first HBV vaccine dose within 24 hours of birth.[51] Even fewer were administering HBIG to infants born to mothers infected with HBV. Such data represent a challenge for the goal of HBV elimination because nearly half of all births worldwide are estimated to occur in high HBV-endemic countries.

Box 2
HepB vaccination for adults aged 19 years or older

- Vaccinate any person seeking protection from HBV infection and persons with risk factors for HBV infection with the 3-dose series (http://www.cdc.gov/vaccines/schedules/downloads/adult/adult-combined-schedule.pdf).

- Catch-up
  - Administer missing doses to complete a 3-dose series of HepB vaccine to those persons not vaccinated or not completely vaccinated. The second dose should be administered at least 1 month after the first dose; the third dose should be administered at least 2 months after the second dose (and at least 4 months after the first dose). If the combined hepatitis A and HepB vaccine (Twinrix®) is used, give 3 doses at 0, 1, and 6 months; alternatively, a 4-dose Twinrix® schedule may be used, administered on days 0, 7, and 21 to 30, followed by a booster dose at 12 months.

- Adult patients receiving hemodialysis or with other immunocompromising conditions should receive 1 dose of 40 μg/mL (Recombivax HB®) administered on a 3-dose schedule at 0, 1, and 6 months or 2 doses of 20 μg/mL (Engerix-B®) administered simultaneously on a 4-dose schedule at 0, 1, 2, and 6 months.

At present, there is limited vaccination in low-income and middle-income countries of high-risk adults, particularly susceptible household and sexual contacts of HBsAg-positive persons identified in screening programs.

Current Vaccine Coverage and Impact in the United States

Children
The number of cases of HBV infection has decreased dramatically in the United States because of routine vaccination of infants. A 68% decrease in HBV infection prevalence

---

Box 3
Persons recommended to receive HepB vaccination by risk factor

All infants, children and adolescents

Persons at risk for infection by sexual exposure
- Sex partners of HBsAg-positive persons
- Sexually active persons who are not in a long-term, mutually monogamous relationship (eg, persons with more than 1 sex partner during the previous 6 months)
- Persons seeking evaluation or treatment of a sexually transmitted disease
- Men who have sex with men

Persons at risk for infection by percutaneous or mucosal exposure to blood
- Current or recent injection-drug users
- Household contacts of HBsAg-positive persons
- Residents and staff of facilities for developmentally disabled persons
- Health care and public safety workers with reasonably anticipated risk for exposure to blood or blood-contaminated body fluids
- Persons with end-stage renal disease, including predialysis, hemodialysis, peritoneal dialysis, and home dialysis patients
- Adults with diabetes mellitus who are aged 19 through 59 years

Others
- International travelers to regions with high or intermediate levels (HBsAg prevalence of >2%) of endemic HBV infection
- Persons with chronic liver disease
- Persons with HIV infection
- All other persons seeking protection from HBV infection

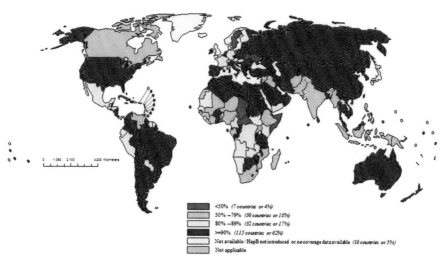

Fig. 1. Immunization coverage with third dose of HepB vaccines in infants, 2014. (*From* WHO/UNICEF coverage estimates 2015 revision. Map production: Immunization Vaccines and Biologicals, (IVB). Geneva: World Health Organization; 2015.)

among US children, regardless of country of origin, was observed within 10 years of initiation of universal hepatitis B vaccination in 1991.[6] Forty-eight perinatal hepatitis B cases were reported.[52] In 2014, vaccination coverage among children aged 19 to 35 months was 91.6% for greater than or equal to 3 doses and 72.4% for the birth dose (1 dose administered by 3 days of life).[53] Vaccine coverage was 91.4% among adolescents age 13–17 years.[54]

High-risk adults

Adult vaccination coverage for hepatitis B in the United States is low. The 2014 National Health Interview Survey reported hepatitis B vaccination coverage (≥3 doses) among adults was 24.5% for adults aged greater than or equal to 19 years, 32.2% among adults aged 19 to 49 years, and 15.7% among adults aged greater than or equal to 50 years.[55] Among adults aged 19 to 49 years, vaccination coverage was lower for black (29.9%) and Hispanic (20.2%) people compared with white people (36.3%). Among high-risk groups, vaccination coverage was 30.5% among adults aged greater than or equal to 19 years who had traveled outside the United States since 1995 to a country in which hepatitis B is of high or intermediate endemicity (regions other than the countries of Europe, Japan, Australia, New Zealand, or Canada); was 29.8% among adults aged greater than or equal to 19 years with chronic liver conditions; and 23.5% for those aged 19 to 59 years with diabetes mellitus (DM). The group with the highest hepatitis B vaccination coverage was health care providers (HCPs); 60.7% overall among HCP aged greater than or equal to 19 years with direct patient care responsibilities (70.9% among white HCPs and 56.6% among black HCPs).

The number of HBV infections among HCPs decreased substantially after hepatitis B vaccine was first recommended for HCPs in 1982 because of the implementation of routine preexposure vaccination and improved infection-control precautions.[56] At present, all unvaccinated persons whose work-related and training-related activities involve reasonably anticipated risk for exposure to blood or other infectious body fluids should be vaccinated with the complete, ≥ 3-dose hepatitis B vaccine series

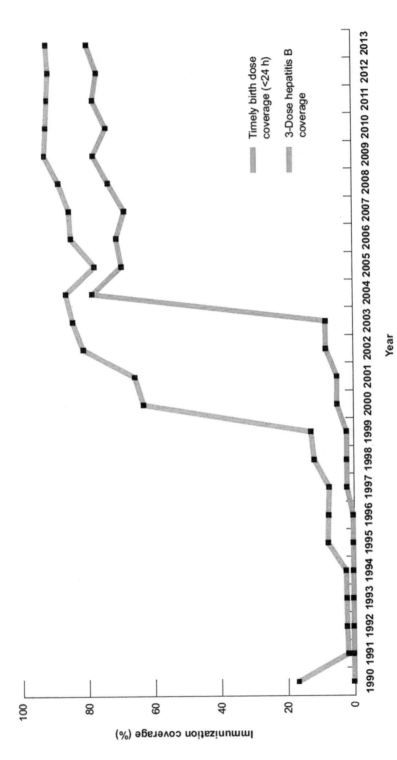

Fig. 2. Immunization coverage with hepatitis B birth dose and third dose, western Pacific region, 1990 to 2013. (*From* World Health Organization. Hepatitis B control through immunization: a reference guide. Geneva: WHO Press, 2014. Available at: http://www.who.int/immunization/sage/meetings/2015/october/8_WPRO_Hepatitis_B_Prevention_Through_Immunization_Regional_Reference_Guide.pdf.)

and undergo postvaccination serologic testing to show protective antibody levels.[57,58]

Hepatitis B vaccination coverage among persons with DM has remained low since the recommendation in 2011 to vaccinate all unvaccinated adults with DM age 19–59 years and adults with DM age $\geq$60 years at the provider's discretion. Infection-control lapses during assisted monitoring of blood glucose levels[32] continue to occur, emphasizing the need to increase hepatitis B vaccination in this population.

Incidence of acute hepatitis B virus infection

Age specific prevalence of HBV vaccine immunity (anti-HBs) was estimated at about 25% of the US non-institutionalized population, based on the last NHANES survey from 2007–2012,[6,9] largely due to routine vaccination policies in newborns, children and adults. Routine vaccination programs in newborns, children, and adults has also had a dramatic effect on reducing the transmission of HBV infection. Routine vaccination has had a dramatic effect on lowering transmission of HBV infection as well. One measure of vaccine impact is the incidence of acute symptomatic HBV in populations. The number of reported cases of acute hepatitis B decreased by 62%, from 8036 in 2000 to 2,953 (0.9/100,000) in 2014 **(Fig. 3)**.[16,52]

Impact of Alaskan vaccination program

In western Alaska, where one of the highest incidences of acute symptomatic HBV infection was found, mass vaccination of susceptible persons coupled with universal vaccination of newborns starting at birth resulted in a dramatic decrease in the annual incidence of acute icteric HBV from more than 200 in 100,000 in 1981 to 0 in 1995, where it has remained.[46,57] The State of Alaska implemented universal infant vaccination for all newborns in 1993, followed by a catch-up vaccination program in children up to 20 years of age, coupled with required proof of HBV vaccination for school entry.

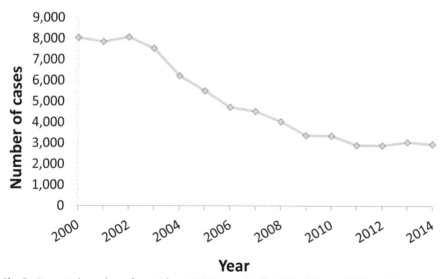

Fig. 3. Reported number of acute hepatitis B cases in the United States, 2000 to 2014. (*From* Centers for Disease Control and Prevention. Viral hepatitis statistics and surveillance. Surveillance for viral hepatitis—United States, 2013. Atlanta (GA): US Department of Health and Human Services; 2015. Available at: http://www.cdc.gov/hepatitis/statistics/2013surveillance/index.htm; with permission.)

The overall incidence of acute HBV in the State of Alaska has decreased to less than 1 in 100,000. In AN children in Alaska, the incidence of acute symptomatic HBV has decreased from 35 in 100,000 in 1983 to 0 in 1993 and no cases have been reported since then.[46] Two countries in which the rates have fallen substantially due to vaccine implementation include Taiwan and Italy. In Taiwan, the incidence of acute symptomatic HBV in children has decreased significantly since the implementation of universal newborn vaccination in the 1980s.[59] In Italy, hepatitis B vaccine was strongly recommended for high risk groups in 1984 and for 3 month olds and 12 years olds in 1991.[60]

Hepatitis B–related Mortality and Liver Cancer

An estimated 39,230 new cases of liver cancer are expected to occur in the United States during 2016; most will be HCC.[61] Chronic infection with HBV or hepatitis C virus is the strongest risk factor for hepatocellular carcinoma, which is the most common type of liver cancer. In the United States, 10% to 15% of patients with HCC are infected with HBV.[62] Prospective cohort studies have shown a 5-fold to 100-fold increase in the risk of developing HCC among persons chronically infected with HBV. However, the age distribution of patients with HCC has shifted to younger ages, with increases among persons 45 to 60 years old. HCC in children is rare.[56] The number and rate of hepatitis B–related deaths overall has been stable for all age group in recent years (2010–2014), at $\leq$0.03 per 100,000 population for persons aged 0 to 34 years and increasing up to 1.8/100,000 in older age groups. In 2014, the overall hepatitis B-related mortality rate was 0.5 deaths/100,000 population (n=1,843).[16]

Incidence of Hepatocellular Carcinoma in Children

Although HCC is not common in children, vaccination programs from Alaska, Taiwan, and Thailand that target newborns and children studies have shown a significant decrease in the incidence of HCC. Before the vaccination campaign in Alaska, the incidence of HCC in children was the highest reported in the world, at 3 per 100,000. Since 1993, no cases of HCC in children caused by HBV have occurred, which is a result of the universal infant and child vaccination program.[63] Furthermore, currently there are no AN children less than 20 years of age in Alaska known to be HBsAg-positive, showing that, with a concerted vaccination program, acute and chronic HBV can be eliminated from a generation. In Taiwan and Thailand, a reduction in the incidence of HCC in children was also shown 10 years after introduction of universal infant vaccination.[64,65]

Hepatocellular Carcinoma in Adults

After the successful implementation of a universal newborn vaccination program followed by a child catch-up program, there will be a several-decade gap before the largest impact on the reduction of the serious sequelae of HBV takes place. The incidence of HCC and decompensated cirrhosis increases slowly in persons infected at birth or early childhood then accelerates exponentially when infected persons reach their late 30s and early 40s. Goldstein and colleagues[36] developed a model to display this graphically (**Fig. 4**). In order to affect the incidence of these serious complications sooner, programs are needed to identify persons infected with HBV, link them to regular care, and intervene with antiviral therapy in those eligible based on current guidelines.[66,67] With currently licensed and recommended antiviral medications (tenofovir and entecavir), HBV cannot be cured, but many new drugs are in clinical development that target different sites in the HBV life cycle and offer potential for a curative strategy.[68]

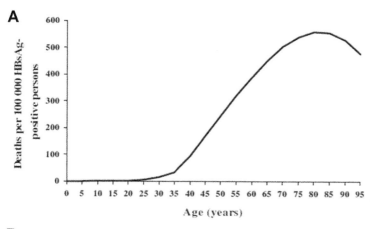

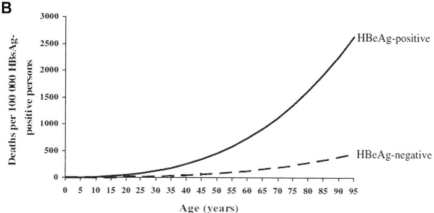

Fig. 4. Mathematical model: age-specific hepatitis B–related cirrhosis (*A*) and HCC (*B*) mortality. (*From* Goldstein ST, Zhou FJ, Hadler SC, et al. A mathematical model to estimate global hepatitis B disease burden and vaccination impact. Int J Epidemiol 2005;34:1329–39; with permission.)

DISCUSSION
Challenges in Implementation of Birth Dose Vaccination in Low-Income and Middle-Income Countries

There are several reasons why many low-resource countries are having difficulty implementing birth dose vaccination within 24 hours of birth. These include:

1. Out-of-hospital births are common in countries with high HBV endemicity, and home deliveries are frequently handled by traditional birth attendants, most of whom have no formal training.
2. In many resource-limited settings, particularly in Africa and Asia, HBV vaccine is only available in a pentavalent preparation (with diphtheria, pertussis, tetanus, and *Haemophilus influenzae* B) and not as a monovalent vaccine for use in newborn babies. The GAVI Alliance (formerly Global Alliance for Vaccines and Immunisation) no longer supports the monovalent vaccine, but only the pentavalent one, which cannot be given in the first 6 weeks of life and is therefore not useful as the birth dose vaccine.

3. Despite extensive evidence that hepatitis B vaccine is extremely safe for neonates and infants, many health care workers still hold misconceptions regarding contra-indications for hepatitis B birth dose vaccination.

Of note, HBIG is also not available or feasible in many low-income countries because its storage requires a cold chain and complex production.[2]

Challenges in Vaccinating Adults at High Risk of Acquiring Hepatitis B Virus as Adults

In the United States, adult vaccination coverage rates are low overall,[62] and this has been attributed to multiple factors, such as limited awareness among the public of the benefit of adult vaccination, inadequate needs assessment for vaccination in adult patient care, payment challenges for patients and providers, and limited stock in health provider offices. Strategies to improve adult immunization in persons at risk for HBV infection and for whom hepatitis B vaccine is recommended include clinical decision support tools, standing orders or protocols for vaccination, and provider and patient reminders. Provider recommendation and convenient access to vaccination are also important.[69]

In the United States, a recent National Academy of Sciences report concluded that control of hepatitis B is feasible, but that eliminating hepatitis B disease will require resources, public support, and addressing barriers.[8] Barriers to elimination identified include surveillance, vaccine tracking, stigma, difficulty reaching foreign-born adults, overworked primary care providers, and need to better understand HBV and management of chronic infection.

Future Goals in Prevention of Mother-to-child Transmission and Vaccination

Some of the key strategies to address current barriers to implementation of the birth dose include the following (summarized in **Box 4**)[49]:

1. Ensuring the provision of monovalent HBV vaccine at an affordable price in low-income countries with high HBV endemicity, which may require further support from GAVI.
2. Storing the HBV vaccine out of the cold chain, which is possible for up to a month (2006 WHO operational field guidelines). The availability of monovalent vaccine in prefilled, single-dose injection devices can also facilitate the administration of the vaccine by birth attendants to infants delivered at home.[70]
3. In addition, collaboration with maternal and child health programs to promote access to skilled birth attendants and postnatal care is critical, together with engagement of community leaders to increase access to available outreach services. Ensuring population confidence in the safety of the vaccine is also important to achieve high vaccine coverage. Education and training of health workers along with communications targeted at the community are needed to address concerns about the timing and safety of administering vaccine immediately after birth and about false contraindications.

The key strategies for control of the HBV epidemic are a combination of universal infant vaccination with three doses of hepatitis B vaccine in the first year of life, together with diagnosis of mothers at high risk of transmitting HBV, those HBeAg-positive or having a level of HBV DNA >200,000 IU/ml in their sera, and use of antiviral agents in the late first or early second trimester to decrease maternal DNA concentrations to undetectable concentrations.

Box 4
Strategies to improve implementation of birth dose and infant vaccination

Service delivery arrangements

- Encourage health-facility deliveries through subsidized deliveries, provide education to mothers during antenatal care, and enhance links with communities.

- Issue standing orders for birth dose vaccination in all health facilities.

- Orientate health and administrative staff on the HBV policy.

- Integrate birth dose with maternal and newborn care in health facilities by:
  ○ Ensuring vaccine is available in the delivery room or postnatal ward
  ○ Establishing clear health-facility policies on where/when/who is to vaccinate
  ○ Positioning birth dose vaccination as part of essential newborn care package
  ○ Providing supportive supervision

- Ensure private facilities provide birth dose vaccination.

- Where infants are born outside health facilities:
  ○ Conduct home visits to provide timely vaccination
  ○ Integrate timely birth dose with home visits for other early postnatal care
  ○ Store vaccine outside the standard cold chain in controlled temperature chain
  ○ Engage village health volunteers to inform health facility of all home births

Health workforce considerations

- Conduct well-structured training for health workers, including education on perinatal transmission, backed up by frequent follow-up and supportive supervision.

Health information system strengthening

- Maintain birth registries and community birth notification, including tracking home births.

- Incorporate birth dose and its timing within vaccination records.

- Use accurate definition of timely birth dose in coverage reporting.

Education

- Address community concerns or lack of knowledge regarding birth dose.

- Address fear of adverse events, including planning for the risk of coincidental newborn death or disease.

- Respond to parental refusal of vaccination.

Data from Practices to improve coverage of the hepatitis B birth dose vaccine. Geneva (Switzerland): World Health Organization; 2012. WHO/IVB/12.11. Available at: http://www.who.int/immunization/documents/control/who_ivb_12.11/en/. Accessed May 13, 2016.

Use of Antiviral Therapy in Women with High Viral Loads

Despite timely administration of HBIG and hepatitis B vaccine starting immediately after birth, 5% to 10% of newborns whose mothers have very high levels of HBV DNA can still acquire HBV infection and develop chronic HBV.[71] Recently, the American Association for the Study of Liver Diseases (AASLD) conducted a systemic review of the evidence that administering antiviral therapy in the third trimester reduces the incidence of HBV transmission to women with very high levels of HBV DNA.[72] From this review, the AASLD, in their updated guideline that used the Grading of Recommendations Assessment, Development and Evaluation (GRADE) approach, recommended that antiviral therapy be administered to HBsAg-positive pregnant mothers in the third trimester whose levels of HBV DNA exceed 200,000 IU/mL[73] but WHO

HBV guidelines have not yet included such a recommendation on use of antiviral therapy.[67] Although lamivudine and telbivudine are both efficacious and considered safe in pregnancy (though long-term safety data are lacking), tenofovir is the drug of choice based on both its potency and high barrier to resistance.

SUMMARY

The hepatitis B vaccine which has been proven to be safe and effective with protection after the vaccine series estimated to persist for at least 30 years among greater than 90% of persons vaccinated,[74] is a key component of chronic hepatitis B prevention and eventual elimination. Routine infant vaccination in over 180 countries has resulted in a reduction in global HBV transmission and declines in chronic HBV prevalence.[1,2] Particular success in reduction of HBV burden from high to low endemicity was achieved in Taiwan and Alaska, US and serve as examples for other areas.[2,75]

Substantial obstacles to global hepatitis B vaccination have been overcome since it was introduced. For example, the cost of vaccine has decreased, the GAVI Alliance has provided targeted assistance to specific countries and implementation of infant immunization programs has broadened.[76] However, many barriers still need to be overcome to achieve elimination of hepatitis B, such as sustained support in developing countries, improved identification of hepatitis B positive mothers, improved implementation of hepatitis B infant vaccination programs including the timely administration of the birth dose, increasing facility-based births to improve access to vaccination, improved cold-chain management for vaccine storage and transport, further exploration of outside the cold chain storage of vaccine,[77] and reducing horizontal transmission among high risk adults. Integrating hepatitis B vaccination with global health initiatives may help sustain existing hepatitis B vaccination programs.[78] Integrating hepatitis B vaccination with screening, care and treatment might also promote general hepatitis B prevention, particularly among pregnant women and is essential for hepatitis B elimination.[60,71]

REFERENCES

1. World Health Organization. Hepatitis B. Available at: www.who.int/topics/hepatitis/factsheets/en. Accessed June 22, 2016.
2. WHO position paper on hepatitis B vaccines - October 2009. Wkly Epidemiol Rec 2009;84:405–20.
3. Schweitzer A, Horn J, Mikolajczyk RT, et al. Estimations of worldwide prevalence of chronic hepatitis B virus infection: a systematic review of data published between 1965 and 2013. Lancet 2015;386(10003):1546–55.
4. GBD 2013 Mortality and Causes of Death Collaborators. Global, regional, and national age-sex specific all-cause and cause-specific mortality for 240 causes of death, 1990-2013: a systematic analysis for the Global Burden of Disease Study 2013. Lancet 2015;385(9963):117–71.
5. Franco E, Bagnato B, Marino MG, et al. Hepatitis B: epidemiology and prevention in developing countries. World J Hepatol 2012;4:74–80.
6. Wasley A, Kruszon-Moran D, Kuhnert W, et al. The prevalence of hepatitis B infection in the United States in the era of vaccination. J Infect Dis 2010;202:192–201.
7. Cohen C, Evans AA, London WT, et al. Underestimation of chronic hepatitis B infection in the United States of America. J Viral Hepat 2008;15:12–3.
8. National Academies of Sciences, Engineering, and Medicine. Eliminating the public health problem of hepatitis B and C in the United States: Phase one report. Washington, DC: The National Academies Press; 2016.

9. Roberts H, Kruszon-Moran D, Ly KN, et al. Prevalence of chronic hepatitis B virus (HBV) infection in U.S. households: National Health and Nutrition Examination Survey (NHANES), 1988-2012. Hepatology 2016;63(2):388–97.

10. Mitchell T, Armstrong GL, Hu DJ, et al. The increasing burden of imported chronic hepatitis B—United States, 1974-2008. PLoS One 2011;6:e27717.

11. Institute of Medicine (US) Committee on the Prevention and Control of Viral Hepatitis Infections, Grossblatt N, editors. Hepatitis and liver cancer: national strategy for prevention and control of hepatitis B and C. Washington, DC: National Academies Press; 2010.

12. Weinbaum CM, Williams I, Mast EE, et al, Centers for Disease Control and Prevention (CDC). Recommendations for identification and public health management of persons with chronic hepatitis B virus infection. MMWR Recomm Rep 2008;57:1–20.

13. Kowdley KV, Wang C, Welch S, et al. Prevalence of chronic hepatitis B among foreign-born persons living in the United States by country of origin. Hepatology 2012;56:422–33.

14. Available at: http://www.cdc.gov/nchs/nhanes/about_nhanes.htm. Accessed August 15, 2016.

15. Centers for Disease Control and Prevention. Asian Americans and hepatitis B. 2013. Available at: http://www.cdc.gov/features/aapihepatitisb/. Accessed May 1, 2015.

16. CDC. Surveillance for viral hepatitis—United States, 2014. Atlanta, GA: US Department of Health and Human Services, CDC; 2014. Available at: http://www.cdc.gov/hepatitis/statistics/2014surveillance/index.htm.

17. Harris AM, Iqbal K, Schillie S, et al. Increases in acute hepatitis B virus infections - Kentucky, Tennessee, and West Virginia, 2006-2013. MMWR Morb Mortal Wkly Rep 2016;65(3):47–50.

18. Centers for Disease Control and Prevention. Update: recommendations to prevent hepatitis B virus transmission-United States. MMWR Morb Mortal Wkly Rep 1995;44:574–5.

19. Edmunds WJ, Medley GF, Nokes DJ, et al. The influence of age on the development of the hepatitis B carrier state. Proc Biol Sci 1993;253:197–201.

20. Hyams KC. Risks of chronicity following acute hepatitis B virus infection: a review. Clin Infect Dis 1995;20:992–1000.

21. Available at: http://www.cdc.gov/hepatitis/Resources/Professionals/PDFs/ABCTable.pdf. Accessed August 15, 2016.

22. Beasley RP, Trepo C, Stevens CE, et al. The e antigen and vertical transmission of hepatitis B surface antigen. Am J Epidemiol 1977;105:94–8.

23. McMahon BJ. Two key components to address chronic hepatitis B in children: detection and prevention. J Pediatr 2015;167:1186–7.

24. Marinier E, Barrois V, Larouze B, et al. Lack of perinatal transmission of hepatitis B virus infection in Senegal, West Africa. J Pediatr 1985;106:843–9.

25. Beasley RP, Hwang LY, Lee GC, et al. Prevention of perinatally transmitted hepatitis B virus infections with hepatitis B virus infections with hepatitis B immune globulin and hepatitis B vaccine. Lancet 1983;2:1099–102.

26. McMahon BJ, Alward WL, Hall DB, et al. Acute hepatitis B virus infection: relation of age to the clinical expression of disease and subsequent development of the carrier state. J Infect Dis 1985;151:599–603.

27. Beasley RP, Hwang LY, Lin CC, et al. Incidence of hepatitis B virus infections in preschool children in Taiwan. J Infect Dis 1982;146:198–204.

28. Coursaget P, Yvonnet B, Chotard J, et al. Age- and sex-related study of hepatitis B virus chronic carrier state in infants from an endemic area (Senegal). J Med Virol 1987;22:1–5.

29. Petersen NJ, Barrett DH, Bond WW, et al. Hepatitis B surface antigen in saliva, impetiginous lesions, and the environment in two remote Alaskan villages. Appl Environ Microbiol 1976;32:572–4.

30. Bond WW, Favero MS, Petersen NJ, et al. Survival of hepatitis B virus after drying and storage for one week. Lancet 1981;1:550–1.

31. Centers for Disease Control and Prevention. Recommendations for preventing transmission of human immunodeficiency virus and hepatitis B virus to patients during exposure-prone invasive procedures. MMWR Recomm Rep 1991; 40(RR-8):1–9.

32. Available at: http://www.cdc.gov/hepatitis/outbreaks/pdfs/healthcareinvestigationtable.pdf. Accessed August 15, 2016.

33. Hepatitis B control through immunization: a reference guide. Available at: http://www.who.int/immunization/sage/meetings/2015/october/8_WPRO_Hepatitis_B_Prevention_Through_Immunization_Regional_Reference_Guide.pdf. Accessed August 15, 2016.

34. Introduction of hepatitis B vaccine into childhood immunization services. Management guidelines, including information for health workers and parents. Available at: http://www.wpro.who.int/hepatitis/whovb0131.pdf. Accessed May 13, 2016.

35. Goldstein ST, Zhou FJ, Hadler SC, et al. A mathematical model to estimate global hepatitis B disease burden and vaccination impact. Int J Epidemiol 2005;34:1329–39.

36. WHO global plan of action on workers' health (2008-2017): baseline for implementation. Available at: http://www.who.int/occupational_health/who_workers_health_web.pdf. Accessed August 15, 2016.

37. Forde KA, Tanapanpanit O, Reddy KR. Hepatitis B and C in African Americans: current status and continued challenges. Clin Gastroenterol Hepatol 2014;12(5):738–48.

38. Mast EE, Margolis HS, Fiore AE, et al. A comprehensive immunization strategy to eliminate transmission of hepatitis B virus infection in the United States: recommendations of the Advisory Committee on Immunization Practices (ACIP) part 1: immunization of infants, children, and adolescents. MMWR Recomm Rep 2005;54:1–31.

39. Schillie S, Murphy TV, Fenlon N, et al. Update: shortened interval for postvaccination serologic testing of infants born to hepatitis B-infected mothers. MMWR Morb Mortal Wkly Rep 2015;64(39):1118–20.

40. Available at: http://www.cdc.gov/vaccines/schedules/index.html. Accessed August 15, 2016.

41. Mast EE, Weinbaum CM, Fiore AE, et al, Advisory Committee on Immunization Practices (ACIP) Centers for Disease Control and Prevention (CDC). A comprehensive immunization strategy to eliminate transmission of hepatitis B virus infection in the United States: recommendations of the Advisory Committee on Immunization Practices (ACIP) Part II: immunization of adults. MMWR Recomm Rep 2006;55(RR-16):1–33 [quiz: CE1–4; Erratum appears in MMWR Morb Mortal Wkly Rep 2007;56(42):1114].

42. Schreeder MT, Bender TR, McMahon BJ, et al. Prevalence of hepatitis B in selected Alaskan Eskimo villages. Am J Epidemiol 1983;118:543–9.

43. Lanier AP, McMahon BJ, Alberts SR, et al. Primary liver cancer in Alaskan natives. 1980-1985. Cancer 1987;60:1915–20.

44. Livingston SE, Simonetti JP, Bulkow LR, et al. Clearance of hepatitis B e antigen in patients with chronic hepatitis B and genotypes A, B, C, D, and F. Gastroenterology 2007;133:1452–7.

45. Heyward WL, Bender TR, McMahon BJ, et al. The control of hepatitis B virus infection with vaccine in Yupik Eskimos. Demonstration of safety, immunogenicity, and efficacy under field conditions. Am J Epidemiol 1985;121:914–23.

46. McMahon BJ, Rhoades ER, Heyward WL, et al. A comprehensive programme to reduce the incidence of hepatitis B virus infection and its sequelae in Alaskan natives. Lancet 1987;2:1134–6.

47. McMahon BJ, Schoenberg S, Bulkow L, et al. Seroprevalence of hepatitis B viral markers in 52,000 Alaska natives. Am J Epidemiol 1993;138:544–9.

48. Peng CY, Chien RN, Liaw YF. Hepatitis B virus-related decompensated liver cirrhosis: benefits of antiviral therapy. J Hepatol 2012 Aug;57(2):442–50.

49. Expanded Programme on Immunization (EPI) of the Department of Immunization, Vaccines and Biologicals. Practices to improve coverage of the hepatitis B birth dose vaccine. Geneva (Switzerland): World Health Organization; 2012. WHO/IVB/12.11. Available at: http://www.who.int/immunization/documents/control/who_ivb_12.11/en/. Accessed May 13, 2016.

50. WHO/UNICEF coverage estimates 2014 revision. 2015. Available at: http://apps.who.int/immunization_monitoring/globalsummary/timeseries/tswucoveragebcg.html. Accessed August 15, 2016.

51. Centers for Disease Control and Prevention (CDC). Global routine vaccination coverage–2012. MMWR Morb Mortal Wkly Rep 2013;62(43):858–61.

52. Adams D, Fullerton K, Jajosky R, et al. Summary of notifiable infectious diseases and conditions - United States, 2013. MMWR Morb Mortal Wkly Rep 2015;62(53):1–122.

53. Hill HA, Elam-Evans LD, Yankey D, et al. National, state, and selected local area vaccination coverage among children aged 19-35 months - United States, 2014. MMWR Morb Mortal Wkly Rep 2015;64(33):889–96.

54. Reagan-Steiner S, Yankey D, Jeyarajah J, et al. National, Regional, State, and Selected Local Area Vaccination Coverage Among Adolescents Aged 13-17 Years–United States, 2014. MMWR Morb Mortal Wkly Rep 2015;64(29):784–92.

55. Williams WW, Lu PJ, O'Halloran A, et al. Surveillance of vaccination coverage among adult populations - United States, 2014. MMWR Surveill Summ 2016;65(1):1–36.

56. Alter MJ, Hadler SC, Margolis HS, et al. The changing epidemiology of hepatitis B in the United States. Need for alternative vaccination strategies. JAMA 1990;263:1218–22.

57. Centers for Disease Control and Prevention. Immunization of health-care personnel: recommendations of the Advisory Committee on Immunization Practices (ACIP). MMWR Recomm Rep 2011;60(RR-7):1–45.

58. Schillie S, Murphy TV, Sawyer M, et al. CDC guidance for evaluating healthcare personnel for hepatitis B virus protection and for administering postexposure management. MMWR Recomm Rep 2013;62(RR-10):1–19.

59. Chien Y-C, Jan C-F, Kuo H-S, et al. Nationwide hepatitis B vaccination program in Taiwan: effectiveness in the 20 years after it was launched. Epidemiol Rev 2006;28:126–35.

60. Stroffolini T, Mele A, Tosti ME, et al. The impact of the hepatitis B mass immunisation campaign on the incidence and risk factors of acute hepatitis B in Italy. J Hepatol 2000;33:980–5.

61. Cancer facts and figures. 2016. Available at: http://www.cancer.org/acs/groups/content/@research/documents/document/acspc-047079.pdf. Accessed August 15, 2016.

62. El-Serag HB. Epidemiology of viral hepatitis and hepatocellular carcinoma. Gastroenterology 2012;142:1264–73.e1.

63. McMahon BJ, Bulkow LR, Singleton RJ, et al. Elimination of hepatocellular carcinoma and acute hepatitis B in children 25 years after a hepatitis B newborn and catch-up immunization program. Hepatology 2011;54:801–7.

64. Wichajarn K, Kosalaraksa P, Wiangnon S. Incidence of hepatocellular carcinoma in children in Khon Kaen before and after National Hepatitis B Vaccine Program. Asian Pac J Cancer Prev 2008;9:507–9.

65. Chang MH, Chen CJ, Lai MS, et al. Universal hepatitis B vaccination in Taiwan and the incidence of hepatocellular carcinoma in children. N Engl J Med 1997;336:1855–9.

66. Terrault NA, Bzowej NH, Chang KM, et al. AASLD guidelines for treatment of chronic hepatitis B. Hepatology 2016;63:261–83.

67. World Health Organization. Guidelines for the prevention, care and treatment of persons with chronic hepatitis B infection. 2015. Available at: http://www.who.int/hiv/pub/hepatitis/hepatitis-b-guidelines/en/. Accessed August 15, 2016.

68. Liang TJ, Block TM, McMahon BJ, et al. Present and future therapies of hepatitis B: from discovery to cure. Hepatology 2015;62:1893–908.

69. Bridges CB, Hurley LP, Williams WW, et al. Meeting the challenges of immunizing adults. Am J Prev Med 2015;49:S455–64.

70. Sutanto A, Suarnawa IM, Nelson CM, et al. Home delivery of heat-stable vaccines in Indonesia: outreach immunization with a prefilled, single-use injection device. Bull World Health Organ 1999;77(2):119–26.

71. Chen HL, Lin LH, Hu FC, et al. Effects of maternal screening and universal immunization to prevent mother-to-infant transmission of HBV. Gastroenterology 2012;142:773–81.e2.

72. Brown RS Jr, McMahon BJ, Lok AS, et al. Antiviral therapy in chronic hepatitis B viral infection during pregnancy: a systematic review and meta-analysis. Hepatology 2016;63:319–33.

73. Terrault NA, Bzowej NH, Chang K, et al. AASLD Guidelines for Treatment of chronic Hepatitis B. Hepatology 2015. Availabe at: https://www.aasld.org/sites/default/files/guideline_documents/hep28156.pdf. Accessed September 7, 2016.

74. Bruce MG, Bruden D, Hurlburt D, et al. Antibody levels and protection after hepatitis B vaccine: results of a 30-year follow-up study and response to a booster dose. J Infect Dis 2016;214(1):16–22.

75. Liang X, Bi S, Yang W, et al. Epidemiological serosurvey of hepatitis B in China–declining HBV prevalence due to hepatitis B vaccination. Vaccine 2009;27(47):6550–7.

76. Hadler SC, Fuqiang C, Averhoff F, et al. The impact of hepatitis B vaccine in China and in the China GAVI Project. Vaccine 2013;31(Suppl 9):J66–72.

77. Kolwaite AR, Xeuatvongsa A, Ramirez-Gonzalez A, et al. Hepatitis B vaccine stored outside the cold chain setting: a pilot study in rural Lao PDR. Vaccine 2016;34(28):3324–30.

78. Van Damme P, Ward J, Shouval D, et al. Hepatitis B vaccines. In: Plotkin S, Orenstein W, Offit P, editors. Vaccines. (China): Saunders; 2012. p. 183–204.

Evolution in Our Understanding of Hepatitis B Virus Virology and Immunology

CrossMark

Bertram Bengsch, MD, PhD[a], Kyong-Mi Chang, MD[b,c],*

KEYWORDS

- Hepatitis B virus • Pathogenesis • Translational hepatology • cccDNA
- Immunobiology • Immunotherapy • B and T cell responses to HBV
- Therapeutic vaccination

KEY POINTS

- Improvements of our understanding of hepatitis B virus (HBV) virology and immunology have been the foundation for the HBV vaccine and current therapies.
- Persistence of cccDNA in HBV-infected hepatocytes represents the major hurdle to cure.
- Immune-based strategies show promise for successful elimination of the reservoir of HBV-infected hepatocytes.

INTRODUCTION

In this article, we first review milestones in the discovery of hepatitis B virus (HBV), its viral cycle and how this led to the development of early diagnostic tests, the understanding of HBV natural history, and the development of HBV vaccines and early therapies. For readers interested in learning about even more details, we highly recommend these excellent recent review articles.[1–3] In the second part of the article, we review the history and limitations of current antiviral therapies, and feature open questions and how recent advances in our understanding of HBV virology and cellular immunology allow for novel rational treatment targets.

Disclosure: Dr. K.-M. Chang has consulting agreements with Arbutus, Alnylam and Genentech. The contents of this work do not represent the views of the Department of Veterans Affairs or the United States Government.
[a] Department of Microbiology and Institute for Immunology, Perelman School of Medicine, University of Pennsylvania, 331 Biomedical Research Building II/III, 421 Curie Boulevard, Philadelphia, PA 19104, USA; [b] Medical Research, Philadelphia Corporal Michael J. Crescenz VA Medical Center (CMC VAMC), A424, University and Woodland Avenue, Philadelphia, PA 19104, USA; [c] Division of Gastroenterology, Department of Medicine, Perelman School of Medicine, University of Pennsylvania, 421 Curie Boulevard, Philadelphia, PA 19104, USA
* Corresponding address. Medical Research, Philadelphia Corporal Michael J. Crescenz VA Medical Center (CMC VAMC), A424, University and Woodland Avenue, Philadelphia PA 19104.
E-mail address: kmchang@mail.med.upenn.edu

IDENTIFICATION OF HEPATITIS B VIRUS

The first descriptions of epidemic jaundice likely owing to viral hepatitis are date back to the times of Hippocrates around 400 BC. In the 19th century, epidemic outbreaks of jaundice several weeks after smallpox vaccination were observed. In seminal work published 1885, Luerman traced the source back to vaccine preparations derived from human "lymph,"[4] suggesting that the epidemic jaundice was caused by an infectious agent, which MacDonald in 1908 proposed to be of viral origin.[5] Further vaccination-associated outbreaks of jaundice occurred during the early part of 20th century, mostly after 1909 and during World War II, associated with the use of hypodermic needles. For example, about 50,000 episodes of jaundice were reported in 1942 among US Army soldiers who received yellow fever vaccine that contained human serum.[6,7] In 1947, MacCallum proposed the term "hepatitis B" for infectious jaundice associated with parenteral transmission route ("serum hepatitis") from "infectious epidemic" hepatitis linked to fecal–oral transmission ("hepatitis A").[8] Subsequent studies conducted in human subjects (often vulnerable populations such as prisoners and mentally handicapped children) showed that hepatitis A and B were likely independent pathogens.[9,10]

The field of viral hepatitis was revolutionized in 1963 by the serendipitous discovery of the HBV surface antigen by Blumberg and Alter. As a geneticist, Baruch Blumberg collected blood samples from different ethnic sources worldwide in an effort to identify polymorphisms involved in certain disease susceptibilities (eg, hemophilia). As Blumberg joined the National Institutes of Health, Harvey Alter was also at the National Institutes of Health studying patients with febrile reactions after blood transfusion, hypothesizing that these reactions may involve antibodies to heterologous serum proteins. Importantly, while performing agar gel immunodiffusion assays with sera from patients with a history of multiple transfusions against samples from Blumberg's collection, Alter identified a reaction against a protein antigen that occurred with high frequency in Australian aborigines. Initially called the 'red antigen' based on its assay appearance, this protein was subsequently named Australia antigen (AuAg).[11] AuAg was subsequently linked to viral hepatitis based on its detection specifically in patients with serum hepatitis.[12–14] These breakthroughs led to the development of diagnostic and screening tests for hepatitis. In 1972, radioimmunoassays replaced first generation agar gel immunodiffusion assays in AuAg detection and contributed to a large reduction in transfusion-associated hepatitis in the 1970s.[2]

However, it was initially difficult to determine if AuAg was the pathogen, a part of the pathogen, or a host protein responding to the pathogen in the absence of established cell culture or animal models that could propagate AuAg. Initial electron microscopy analysis of purified AuAg by Blumberg and colleagues[15] identified small round particles of variable size (15–25 nm) that seemed different from known viruses and did not seem to contain nucleic acids by the experimental approaches used then. These observations even led to the speculation that AuAg might be a prionlike agent. However, subsequent electron microscopy studies of AuAg immunocomplexes by David S. Dane showed that AuAg was also incorporated into larger particles with an inner core structure.[16] Recognition of isolated core protein (HBcAg) by patient antibodies[17] suggested that the Dane particles represented the actual HBV, the AuAg being its surface protein (HBsAg). DNA polymerase activity and double-stranded DNA molecules in purified AuAg preparations then showed that the Dane particles contained intact HBV with a nucleic acid genome.[18,19] The HBV DNA was subsequently cloned and elicited acute HBV infection after injection into chimpanzee livers,[20] demonstrating that the Dane particles indeed represented infectious HBV.

THE DEVELOPMENT AND SUCCESS OF THE VACCINE

Passive immunization strategies against HBV, using sera from immune patients, are effective shortly after exposure or against perinatal transmission. However, the protective effects are only transient owing to the short half-life of the transferred antibodies.[21] Accordingly, the discovery of the HBsAg provided a rational target for a vaccine antigen. Small (eg, putatively HBV DNA-free) HBsAg particles were isolated from patient plasma, further purified and inactivated before use as a vaccine with extensive testing in chimpanzees (first vaccination attempts with crudely inactivated AuAg preparations performed in mentally impaired children were discontinued owing to ethical concerns).[22] The HBsAg preparations were highly protective against infection with a potent antibody response[23,24] and subsequently used to vaccinate health care professionals and other high-risk populations.[25,26] However, the approach to use isolated HBsAg particles from patients was not without risks, including those related to infectious agents such as human immunodeficiency virus (HIV) and hepatitis C virus. The successful cloning of the HBV genome and identification of the HBs gene allowed for a recombinant gene technology approach; after expression of HBsAg in *Escherichia coli* was initially unsuccessful, yeast strains were generated that expressed HBsAg and allowed large-scale production at a low cost. The recombinant vaccine proved highly protective in chimpanzees and humans[27,28] and was adopted as the standard vaccine recommended by the World Health Organization. Importantly, in populations with a high HBV prevalence, such as Taiwan, introduction of the HBV vaccine rapidly reduced perinatal HBV transmission, and long-term reduced incidence of HCC.[29,30] Thus, HBsAg vaccine is likely to be the single most effective preventive anticancer agent.

THE HEPATITIS B VIRUS PROTEINS AND THEIR RELATIONSHIP TO THE NATURAL HISTORY OF HEPATITIS B VIRUS INFECTION

The successful cloning of the HBV DNA revealed the unique small open circular viral DNA with overlapping open reading frames encoding HBsAg, HBcAg, the DNA polymerase and an additional "X" gene.[19,31–33] Interestingly, Magnius and Espmark[34] discovered an additional, "enigmatic antigen," "HBeAg," that was prevalent in highly infectious HBsAg-positive samples, but not in HBsAg-positive samples with low infectivity. Later, the HBeAg was identified as protein variant of HBcAg that is produced depending on a signal sequence preceding the HBc gene.[35,36] The serologic testing for HBV antigens provided a framework to distinguish different clinical phases of HBV infection. For example, emergence of anti-HBsAg and loss of HBsAg indicated viral clearance after acute infection, whereas persistent HBsAg is the hallmark of chronic HBV infection. Chronic HBV infection was initially divided into 2 phases: an initial HBeAg-positive phase with active liver disease and viral replication and an HBeAg-negative healthy carrier phase without liver disease or viral replication.[37] This evolved to 3 phases that included an immune-tolerant phase with high-level viremia without biochemical or histologic evidence of liver inflammation. With improved detection of HBV DNA through[37] polymerase chain reaction in 1990s, active HBV viremia was identified in some HBeAg-negative HBsAg-positive patients. In addition, a subset of HBsAg-negative subjects displayed 'occult' hepatitis B with detectable HBV DNA and variable clinical and/or immunologic significance.[38–40]

The immune response is believed to play a key role in the outcome of HBV infection. Although the precise underlying mechanisms for liver disease pathogenesis are not defined clearly, the levels of hepatitis and viral replication observed in various phases of chronic hepatitis B are thought to reflect distinct states of virus–host immune interactions. Typically, vertical HBV transmission from mother to neonate is associated initially with an immune tolerant phase with HBeAg status and high levels of viral replication without any liver enzyme elevation. After 1 to 2 decades, this phase may change to an HBeAg-positive immune active phase with increased alanine aminotransferase levels and fluctuating viral load that can convert into an HBeAg-negative inactive carrier phase characterized by low levels of viral replication and low alanine aminotransferase. A subset of HBeAg-negative patients show fluctuating alanine aminotransferase and necroinflammatory liver disease (either owing to HBV reactivation after variable duration of inactive carrier state or directly from HBeAg-positive chronic hepatitis).[37]

HEPATITIS B VIRUS AND THE RISK FOR HEPATOCELLULAR CARCINOMA

The development of HBV serologic detection assays enabled epidemiologic studies identifying chronic hepatitis B as a significant risk factor for hepatocellular carcinoma (HCC).[41] For example, HCC was the most frequent cancer in areas with high prevalence of chronic HBV infection, such as in Taiwan. Furthermore, risk of HCC was dramatically increased by 223-fold among chronic HBsAg carriers in a study of 22,707 Chinese men in Taiwan, whereas HCC and cirrhosis accounted for 54% of 105 deaths in HBsAg carriers compared with only 1.5% among 202 deaths in noncarriers.[42] The cellular mechanisms driving the oncogenicity of HBV, however, are complex and less understood. The integration of HBV DNA fragments into the genome of HCCs has been frequently observed, suggesting that HBV proteins might be directly oncogenic. Since several HBV DNA elements (eg, preS/S and X proteins) may act as transcriptional activators, overexpression and/or integration of these proteins may contribute to prooncogenic transcriptional programs.[43–45] In addition, random integration of HBV DNA in the genomic DNA may activate cellular oncogenes or disrupt proliferation checkpoints. Interestingly, some insertions may result in chimeric HBV fusion transcripts that regulate microRNA activity, epigenetically promoting HCC development.[46,47] However, insertions of HBV elements into the DNA seem to be random, which argues against a common mechanism of HCC development in HBV-related HCC. In addition, occurrence of most HCCs in patients with advanced liver cirrhosis suggest a pathogenetic role for altered liver microenvironment and immune surveillance in the cirrhotic liver.

CURRENT ANTIVIRAL THERAPIES
Interferon

Shortly after the discovery of HBsAg, treatment with interferon (IFN)-α was shown to suppress HBV replication and cure patients with chronic HBV infection.[48] However, further follow-up and improvements in diagnostics clarified that most patients relapse after treatment cessation and that viral clearance is rare. Despite the low cure rates, IFN therapy may promote a seroconversion from the highly viremic HBeAg-positive phase to a low viremic HBeAg-negative phase of infection by stimulating endogenous immune responses (particularly in patients with liver inflammation and moderate viremia), suggesting a benefit with long-term virus control. Although IFN therapy is challenging owing to its side effects and parenteral administration compared with oral nucleoside or nucleotide analogs (NUCs), the use of IFN is being reconsidered in combination with NUCs owing to greater cure rates with loss of HBsAg.[49]

NUCLEOSIDE AND NUCLEOTIDE ANALOGS

HBV DNA recovered from serum viral particles was found to be significantly different from other DNA viruses in that its circular DNA contained noncovalently closed DNA strands of unequal length complexed with protein.[19,50] Moreover, HBV DNA polymerase displayed a reverse transcriptase function.[51] Hence, HBV replicates by first transcribing an RNA template that is then converted into a DNA strand, with significant mechanistic similarities to retroviral replication.[52] After release into hepatocytes, the incomplete HBV DNA is repaired in the nucleus by cellular repair enzymes and establishes a pool of covalently closed circular HBV DNA (cccDNA) that serves as template for cellular RNA polymerase II, which generates pregenomic and subgenomic messenger RNAs. The viral polymerase localizes with the viral RNA to the viral core particle and initiates reverse transcription.

Among nucleoside or nucleotide inhibitors of HIV reverse transcriptase, lamivudine was the first NUC to show clinical success in suppressing HBV replication in HIV-coinfected and monoinfected patients.[53,54] Although lamivudine treatment was well-tolerated and resulted in rapid improvement of liver disease with subsequent reduction in viral titers, it did not eliminate the HBV cccDNA and rapidly selected for resistant HBV variants with mutations in the reverse transcriptase domain of the HBV DNA polymerase. These findings prompted the development of new NUCs with more favorable resistance profiles (eg, adefovir and telbivudine). However, resistance remained a significant clinical problem until the introduction of entecavir and tenofovir, which are both highly potent with long-term resistance rates of close to 0%.[55] Thus, entecavir and tenofovir have emerged as a major treatment regimen for chronic hepatitis B. However, unfortunately, NUC therapy does not eliminate viral cccDNA and recurrent viremia is the rule upon treatment cessation in most patients.[56] Furthermore, although combination therapies of NUCs with IFN are associated with increased cure rates with HBsAg loss compared with NUC alone, absolute rates of HBV elimination remain low.[49] Despite the great success of NUC therapies, these problems highlight the need for novel therapeutic approaches.

HEPATITIS B VIRUS ENTRY INHIBITORS

The primary HBV receptor remained elusive until 2012, when the liver-specific sodium-dependent taurochlorate cotransporting polypeptide, a bile acid transporter, was identified to be bound by the pre-S1 domain of the large envelope protein and required for HBV cellular entry.[57] Compounds that inhibit HBV–sodium-dependent taurochlorate cotransporting polypeptide interaction, such as myrcludex-B, a synthetic lipopeptide consisting of the myristoylated 2 to 48 aa region of preS1, are able to strongly inhibit HBV infection in preclinical models and are currently investigated in clinical trials.[58,59] Of note, this compound may be efficacious against HBV (and hepatitis D virus) at concentrations that permit transport of physiologic targets (eg, bile salts), suggesting a favorable side effect profile.[60] This may not hold true for other compounds that target sodium-dependent taurochlorate cotransporting polypeptide and reduce HBV entry, such as cyclosporine, a well-characterized calcineurin inhibitor generally used as an immunosuppressive agent.[61]

STRATEGIES TARGETING HEPATITIS B VIRUS COVALENTLY CLOSED CIRCULAR DNA

The persistence of the nuclear HBV cccDNA as an episomal minichromosome remains the major challenge for HBV elimination.

The use of genetically modified enzymes of the CRISPR/Cas9 RNA-guided nuclease system has enabled researchers to selectively target genomic DNA and specifically cut DNA based on an RNA guiding template. Direct targeting of HBV cccDNA sequences with this technology may be a direct way to attack the viral genome within the nucleus. Several recent reports have used this strategy and designed guides for HBV sequences that were effective in disrupting episomal cccDNA and chromosomally integrated HBV, consequently disrupting HBV replication.[62–65] Despite promising results and convincing rationale, safety concerns arising from genome editing of host DNA independent of the HBV genome remain, because current CRISPR/Cas9 approaches are known for low frequency but significant off-target cleavage and recombination events.

As a part of innate immunity, cytidine deaminases of the APOBEC family also target viral genomes and may inhibit viral replication by genome editing. Members of the APOBEC3 subfamily were found to interfere with HBV replication, a mechanism that seems to be evaded by the virus in chronic infection.[66–68] Recently, however, Lucifora and colleagues[69] described how members of the APOBEC3 family can be induced downstream of IFN and lymphotoxin receptor signaling to degrade HBV cccDNA in hepatocytes, highlighting the antiviral effect of innate cellular immune defense mechanisms. Importantly, no editing of the host genome was observed in the study. Thus, although the experimental strategies used in these studies might invoke systemic side effects, it may be possible to develop compounds that induce similar APOBEC3 activity that are better suited for combination therapies with NUCs. Moreover, they also highlight the potential use of host immune defense mechanisms for clearance of HBV infection.

HARNESSING THE IMMUNE SYSTEM TO ELIMINATE HEPATITIS B VIRUS INFECTION

The adaptive immune system is critical in the elimination and pathophysiology of HBV infection. The liver damage in acute clinical hepatitis is related to immune cell infiltrates and thought to be secondary to adaptive immune responses. Although HBV may represent a "stealth virus" that initially does not induce innate immune response for several weeks, HBV is cleared as adaptive immune responses are induced.[70] Successful immune responses in acute resolving HBV infection may provide a rational framework to identify critical components of effective antiviral immunity.

INNATE IMMUNE RESPONSES

Innate immunity is the first line of defense against pathogens. Recognition of pathogen-associated molecular patterns through innate pattern recognition receptors (eg, toll-like receptors or other intracellular sensors) induces antiviral gene programs, including IFN and IFN-stimulated genes, with direct and indirect antiviral effects. In addition, innate immune cells, such as neutrophils, macrophages, innate lymphoid cells, natural killer (NK) cells, NK T cells, and dendritic cells are activated to produce cytokines and chemokines that can recruit other immune cells with inflammatory as well as antiviral effects. Innate immune activation is also critical in the development of adaptive immune responses.

Remarkably, HBV is transcriptionally silent in acute infection, with little to no induction of host innate response (including IFN-inducible genes), in stark contrast to hepatitis C virus, which induces numerous IFN-inducible genes in chimpanzee model of experimental HBV infection.[70,71] Similarly, type I IFN is barely detectable in acutely HBV-infected patients.[72] These in vivo findings suggested that HBV is a 'stealth virus' that bypasses the innate sensing machinery during early infection. Furthermore, HBV is readily suppressed by innate immune components including IFN-α,[49,73] toll-like receptor, NK, NK T cells, and antigen-presenting cells.[74] Nevertheless, additional studies suggest that innate immune cells are activated and contribute to the course of acute[75–77] and chronic HBV infection.[78–82] Because acute HBV infection is mostly resolved in otherwise healthy adults, the early innate immune evasion by HBV may be important for the initial establishment of infection, rather than persistence of HBV infection. Moreover, depletion studies in chimpanzees suggest that the actual elimination of HBV infection requires the presence of adaptive immune responses.

In addition to initiating adaptive immune responses, innate immunity may be intricately involved in cooperation with adaptive immune functions. For example, platelets are required for optimal intrahepatic T-cell immunosurveillance with the potential to aggravate hepatitis.[81,82] In chronic infection, however, innate immune responses may contribute to an immunosuppressive microenvironment with potential pathogenetic effects. For example, NK cells from patients with chronic hepatitis B display altered phenotype and function.[78,79] Along these lines, dendritic cells from patients with chronic hepatitis B showed higher levels of activation with impaired capacity to induce NK cell effector function.[83,84] Furthermore, hepatitis flares during chronic hepatitis B coincided with increased serum IFN-α levels, NK activation and expression of tumor necrosis factor-related apoptosis inducing ligand (TRAIL).[85] Interestingly, NK cells may eliminate HBV-specific T cells by a TRAIL-mediated mechanism[80] whereas myeloid-derived suppressor cells may accumulate in chronic infections and metabolically regulate effector responses.[86] Thus, HBV may initially evade innate immune recognition to establish infection. However, multiple innate immune pathways are ultimately induced in acute and chronic HBV infection with relevance to clinical outcome.

B CELLS

The B-cell antibody response to the HBsAg is the major correlate of vaccination success, suggesting that B cells play an important role in the immune response to HBV infection. In patients with serologically resolved HBV infection, B-cell depletion owing to cancer therapies may result in HBV reactivation, suggesting an active role for B cells in viral control.[87] However, in chronic HBV infection, the virus persists despite high levels of virus-specific antibodies being present.[88] The link between characteristic antibody response patterns and the immunologic phases of HBV suggests a link of B-cell responses to the natural history of infection. However, our understanding of the mechanisms behind these associations is limited. The excessive production of defective HBV virions serving as decoys is thought to contribute to HBV escape from the B cell response. Moreover, the abundance of antibodies produced may cause accumulation of immune complexes that can drive significant pathology, such as in extrahepatic manifestations of HBV (eg, HBV-associated glomerulonephritis). Interestingly, IL-10–producing B cells have been described in chronic HBV infection and their accumulation was associated with peak hepatitis flares.[89] Depletion of B cells in vitro enhanced the antiviral T-cell response, suggesting that B cells may acquire regulatory functions during chronic HBV infection.[89] Further studies are required to elucidate the role of HBV-specific B cells during chronic HBV infection.

T CELLS

As early as 1977, T-cell infiltrates were noted as the dominant immune cell subset infiltrating the liver in acute hepatitis B infection.[90] In the early 1990s, identification of multiple T-cell epitopes within the HBV genome helped identify HBV-specific cell responses that were associated with viral clearance.[91–95] Advances in technology revealed a tight correlation of HBV-specific effector T-cell responses during the acute phase with clearance of infection.[96] In the chimpanzee model of HBV infection, depletion studies of CD8[+] and CD4[+] T cells revealed a requirement of CD8[+] T cells for the elimination of HBV infection,[97] whereas CD4 T-cell responses seem to be required for CD8 T-cell support. CD8[+] T cells are able to eliminate virus in infected cells by cytolytic and noncytolytic pathways. T cells may induce killing of infected cells by the release of pore-forming perforin and apoptosis-inducing granzyme proteases into the target cell or the engagement of surface death receptors. Despite the link of T cells to the liver damage in hepatitis, the majority of the antiviral effect of HBV-specific T cells is attributed to noncytolytic pathways. Secretion of antiviral cytokines (eg, IFN-γ, tumor necrosis factor) is thought to be key to noncytolytic elimination of virus in infected cells.[98] Interestingly, the onset of viral clearance in HBV-infected chimpanzees is closely correlated with intrahepatic accumulation of IFN-γ–producing CD8[+] T cells, preceding the peak of liver damage.[99] During acute resolving infection, a pool of phenotypic and functional memory T cells is established that is thought to provide protection upon rechallenge.[100] In sum, these studies indicate that HBV-specific CD8[+] T cells are key to the elimination of HBV during acute infection.

Immune Regulation of T-Cell Effector Responses

However, during chronic HBV infection, HBV-specific CD8[+] T cells remain detectable at lower frequencies compared with acute infection and an exhaustion of antiviral T-cell responses is observed.[101–103] HBV-specific T cells in chronic infection are found to express inhibitory receptors, such as PD-1, that contribute to reduced proliferation and cytokine production.[104] The PD-1 pathway is of interest, since therapeutic interventions blocking PD-1 signaling are efficient strategies to improve T-cell responses in other chronic viral infections and cancer.[105] In agreement with this notion, intrahepatic HBV-specific T-cell responses can be improved by PD-1 blockade in vitro.[106] This effect can be enhanced by additional application of costimulatory signals, such as by stimulation of the receptor 4-1BB.[107] Exhausted T cells, however, may express multiple inhibitory receptors and coexpression of inhibitory receptors may confer additional inhibitory signals. Strategies to block other inhibitory receptors, such as CTLA-4, Tim-3 or BTLA, may be required to enhance HBV-specific effector function.[108–110] However, the identification of optimal inhibitory receptor blockade strategies may require a detailed analysis of the T-cell differentiation state and phase of chronic infection.[111] Of note, the inhibitory receptors upregulated by HBV-specific T cells are also involved in the tolerogenic function of the liver.[112] Targeting of these inhibitory pathways in settings of viral infection may desirably enhance antiviral effector function but could also cause significant collateral damage, which may be relevant since up to 100% of hepatocytes can be infected with HBV. In animal models, absence of the inhibitory receptor PD-1 caused fulminant hepatitis in adenoviral infection.[113] However, anecdotal reports of PD-1 blockade strategies in cancer patients coinfected with HBV suggest a favorable safety profile.[114]

In addition to inhibitory receptors, several mechanisms have been implicated in the induction of exhausted T-cell responses. These include limited CD4[+] helper T-cell responses,[115,116] induction of regulatory T cells that suppress CD8[+] T cells,[117] induction of T-cell proapoptotic factors (eg, Bim),[118] a suppressive rather than supportive cytokine milieu[89,116,119] and metabolic regulation of the liver environment, such as by depletion of critical amino acids required for T-cell metabolism in the inflamed liver environment,[120,121] which may be related to the activity of myeloid-derived suppressor cells.[86] In contrast, even though viral evasion of T-cell responses by selection of escape mutations has been described in HBV, the impact of viral escape in HBV is thought to be small compared with other viral infections.[122]

Although these mechanistic insights characterize rational targets for immunomodulatory therapies, they also highlight the complexity of the immune interactions during chronic HBV infection.

Therapeutic Vaccination

The protective HBsAg-based vaccine successful in inducing protective immunity in uninfected subjects is unfortunately ineffective during chronic infection,[123] although induction of adaptive immune responses can be observed in some patients and in settings of NUC coadministration.[124] Because protein antigens, such as HBsAg, may induce B cell and CD4$^+$ T-cell responses rather than CD8$^+$ T-cell responses, which are thought to be the cell subset required to clear infected hepatocytes, vaccination efforts with peptides representing CD8$^+$ T-cell epitopes have been tested. A study used an immunodominant HBV epitope to induce vaccine responses and showed immunogenicity, however, the vaccination failed to significantly impact on HBV viral titers.[125] It is likely that inclusion of multiple T-cell epitopes into a vaccine would be required for therapeutic response. The approach to vaccinate with multiple HBV proteins by using DNA vaccination strategies showed some promise when combined with NUC therapy and IL-12 coadministration, but did not achieve a significant effect on HBV DNA suppression in a larger study.[126,127] It is possible that the unsatisfying results from the vaccination trials stem from the focus of targeting specific arms of the immune response with consensus virus proteins. In a recent study, Gehring and colleagues[128] suggested the possibility to harness patient monocyte populations for the presentation of personalized HBV antigens, which might overcome some barriers to vaccination success by activating multiple arms of the immune system to relevant antigens.

Genetically Modified T Cells

In addition to reinvigoration strategies of functionally impaired antiviral T cells, therapeutic vaccination, infusion of genetically modified HBV-specific T cells expanded in vitro represents an interesting therapeutic concept. By inducing fully functional T-cell responses in vitro, the modified T cells may be more resistant to the immunoregulatory environment virus-specific T cells face in chronic HBV, endowing them with the ability to overcome the T-cell failure in chronic HBV. Transduction of endogenous T cells with a chimeric antigen receptor specific for the tumor antigen and subsequent adoptive transfer has been a breakthrough in several difficult-to-treat cancers.[129] HBV-specific CARs targeting the HBV envelope proteins show antiviral efficiency in animal models,[130] providing a proof of principle for the application of CAR therapies in HBV infection.

REFERENCES

1. Alter HJ. The road not taken or how I learned to love the liver: a personal perspective on hepatitis history. Hepatology 2014;59:4–12.
2. Gerlich WH. Medical virology of hepatitis B: how it began and where we are now. Virol J 2013;10:239.
3. Thomas E, Yoneda M, Schiff ER. Viral hepatitis: past and future of HBV and HDV. Cold Spring Harb Perspect Med 2015;5:a021345.
4. Luerman A. Eine icterusepidemie. Ber Klin Wochenschr 1885;20–3.
5. McDonald S. Acute yellow atrophy. Edinb Med J 1908;15:108.

6. Seeff LB, Beebe GW, Hoofnagle JH, et al. A serologic follow-up of the 1942 epidemic of post-vaccination hepatitis in the United States Army. N Engl J Med 1987;316:965–70.

7. Martin NA. The discovery of viral hepatitis: a military perspective. J R Army Med Corps 2003;149:121–4.

8. MacCallum FO. Homologous serum jaundice. Lancet 1947;2:691–2.

9. Krugman S, Giles JP, Hammond J. Infectious hepatitis. Evidence for two distinctive clinical, epidemiological, and immunological types of infection. JAMA 1967;200:365–73.

10. Melnick JL, Boggs JD. Human volunteer and tissue culture studies of viral hepatitis. Can Med Assoc J 1972;106(Suppl):461–7.

11. Blumberg BS, Alter HJ, Visnich S. A "new" antigen in leukemia sera. JAMA 1965;191:541–6.

12. Blumberg BS, Gerstley BJ, Hungerford DA, et al. A serum antigen (Australia antigen) in Down's syndrome, leukemia, and hepatitis. Ann Intern Med 1967;66:924–31.

13. Okochi K, Murakami S. Observations on Australia antigen in Japanese. Vox Sang 1968;15:374–85.

14. Prince AM. An antigen detected in the blood during the incubation period of serum hepatitis. Proc Natl Acad Sci U S A 1968;60:814–21.

15. Blumberg BS. The discovery of the hepatitis B virus and the invention of the vaccine: a scientific memoir. J Gastroenterol Hepatol 2002;17(Suppl):S502–3.

16. Dane DS, Cameron CH, Briggs M. Virus-like particles in serum of patients with Australia-antigen-associated hepatitis. Lancet 1970;1:695–8.

17. Almeida JD, Rubenstein D, Stott EJ. New antigen-antibody system in Australia-antigen-positive hepatitis. Lancet 1971;2:1225–7.

18. Robinson WS, Clayton DA, Greenman RL. DNA of a human hepatitis B virus candidate. J Virol 1974;14:384–91.

19. Robinson WS, Greenman RL. DNA polymerase in the core of the human hepatitis B virus candidate. J Virol 1974;13:1231–6.

20. Will H, Cattaneo R, Koch HG, et al. Cloned HBV DNA causes hepatitis in chimpanzees. Nature 1982;299:740–2.

21. Beasley RP, Hwang LY, Lin CC, et al. Hepatitis B immune globulin (HBIG) efficacy in the interruption of perinatal transmission of hepatitis B virus carrier state. Initial report of a randomised double-blind placebo-controlled trial. Lancet 1981;2:388–93.

22. Krugman S, Giles JP, Hammond J. Viral hepatitis, type B (MS-2 strain) prevention with specific hepatitis B immune serum globulin. JAMA 1971;218:1665–70.

23. Hilleman MR, Buynak EB, Roehm RR, et al. Purified and inactivated human hepatitis B vaccine: progress report. Am J Med Sci 1975;270:401–4.

24. Purcell RH, Gerin JL. Hepatitis B subunit vaccine: a preliminary report of safety and efficacy tests in chimpanzees. Am J Med Sci 1975;270:395–9.

25. Maupas P, Goudeau A, Coursaget P, et al. Immunisation against hepatitis B in man. Lancet 1976;1:1367–70.

26. Szmuness W, Stevens CE, Harley EJ, et al. Hepatitis B vaccine: demonstration of efficacy in a controlled clinical trial in a high-risk population in the United States. N Engl J Med 1980;303:833–41.

27. McAleer WJ, Buynak EB, Maigetter RZ, et al. Human hepatitis B vaccine from recombinant yeast. Nature 1984;307:178–80.

28. Poovorawan Y, Sanpavat S, Pongpunlert W, et al. Protective efficacy of a recombinant DNA hepatitis B vaccine in neonates of HBe antigen-positive mothers. JAMA 1989;261:3278–81.

29. Chang MH, You SL, Chen CJ, et al. Decreased incidence of hepatocellular carcinoma in hepatitis B vaccinees: a 20-year follow-up study. J Natl Cancer Inst 2009;101:1348–55.

30. Poovorawan Y, Chongsrisawat V, Theamboonlers A, et al. Evidence of protection against clinical and chronic hepatitis B infection 20 years after infant vaccination in a high endemicity region. J Viral Hepat 2011;18:369–75.

31. Charnay P, Pourcel C, Louise A, et al. Cloning in Escherichia coli and physical structure of hepatitis B virion DNA. Proc Natl Acad Sci U S A 1979;76:2222–6.

32. Pasek M, Goto T, Gilbert W, et al. Hepatitis B virus genes and their expression in E. coli. Nature 1979;282:575–9.

33. Valenzuela P, Gray P, Quiroga M, et al. Nucleotide sequence of the gene coding for the major protein of hepatitis B virus surface antigen. Nature 1979;280:815–9.

34. Magnius LO, Espmark A. A new antigen complex co-occurring with Australia antigen. Acta Pathol Microbiol Scand B Microbiol Immunol 1972;80:335–7.

35. Bruss V, Gerlich WH. Formation of transmembraneous hepatitis B e-antigen by cotranslational in vitro processing of the viral precore protein. Virology 1988;163:268–75.

36. Standring DN, Ou JH, Masiarz FR, et al. A signal peptide encoded within the precore region of hepatitis B virus directs the secretion of a heterogeneous population of e antigens in Xenopus oocytes. Proc Natl Acad Sci U S A 1988;85:8405–9.

37. Yim HJ, Lok AS. Natural history of chronic hepatitis B virus infection: what we knew in 1981 and what we know in 2005. Hepatology 2006;43:S173–81.

38. Raimondo G, Pollicino T, Romano L, et al. A 2010 update on occult hepatitis B infection. Pathol Biol (Paris) 2010;58:254–7.

39. Lok AS, Everhart JE, Di Bisceglie AM, et al. Occult and previous hepatitis B virus infection are not associated with hepatocellular carcinoma in United States patients with chronic hepatitis C. Hepatology 2011;54:434–42.

40. Rehermann B, Ferrari C, Pasquinelli C, et al. The hepatitis B virus persists for decades after patients' recovery from acute viral hepatitis despite active maintenance of a cytotoxic T-lymphocyte response. Nat Med 1996;2:1104–8.

41. Szmuness W, Stevens CE, Ikram H, et al. Prevalence of hepatitis B virus infection and hepatocellular carcinoma in Chinese-Americans. J Infect Dis 1978;137:822–9.

42. Beasley RP, Hwang LY, Lin CC, et al. Hepatocellular carcinoma and hepatitis B virus. A prospective study of 22 707 men in Taiwan. Lancet 1981;2:1129–33.

43. Hohne M, Schaefer S, Seifer M, et al. Malignant transformation of immortalized transgenic hepatocytes after transfection with hepatitis B virus DNA. EMBO J 1990;9:1137–45.

44. Kekule AS, Lauer U, Meyer M, et al. The preS2/S region of integrated hepatitis B virus DNA encodes a transcriptional transactivator. Nature 1990;343:457–61.

45. Lucifora J, Arzberger S, Durantel D, et al. Hepatitis B virus X protein is essential to initiate and maintain virus replication after infection. J Hepatol 2011;55:996–1003.

46. Lau CC, Sun T, Ching AK, et al. Viral-human chimeric transcript predisposes risk to liver cancer development and progression. Cancer Cell 2014;25:335–49.

47. Liang HW, Wang N, Wang Y, et al. Hepatitis B virus-human chimeric transcript HBx-LINE1 promotes hepatic injury via sequestering cellular microRNA-122. J Hepatol 2016;64:278–91.

48. Greenberg HB, Pollard RB, Lutwick LI, et al. Effect of human leukocyte interferon on hepatitis B virus infection in patients with chronic active hepatitis. N Engl J Med 1976;295(10):517–22.

49. Marcellin P, Ahn SH, Ma X, et al. Combination of tenofovir disoproxil fumarate and peginterferon alpha-2a increases loss of hepatitis B surface antigen in patients with chronic hepatitis B. Gastroenterology 2016;150:134–44.e10.

50. Gerlich WH, Robinson WS. Hepatitis B virus contains protein attached to the 5' terminus of its complete DNA strand. Cell 1980;21:801–9.

51. Summers J, Mason WS. Replication of the genome of a hepatitis B–like virus by reverse transcription of an RNA intermediate. Cell 1982;29:403–15.

52. Nassal M. Hepatitis B viruses: reverse transcription a different way. Virus Res 2008;134:235–49.

53. Benhamou Y, Dohin E, Lunel-Fabiani F, et al. Efficacy of lamivudine on replication of hepatitis B virus in HIV-infected patients. Lancet 1995;345:396–7.

54. Dienstag JL, Perrillo RP, Schiff ER, et al. A preliminary trial of lamivudine for chronic hepatitis B infection. N Engl J Med 1995;333:1657–61.

55. Zoulim F. Hepatitis B virus resistance to antiviral drugs: where are we going? Liver Int 2011;31(Suppl 1):111–6.

56. Terrault NA, Bzowej NH, Chang KM, et al. AASLD guidelines for treatment of chronic hepatitis B. Hepatology 2016;63:261–83.

57. Yan H, Zhong G, Xu G, et al. Sodium taurocholate cotransporting polypeptide is a functional receptor for human hepatitis B and D virus. Elife 2012;1:e00049.

58. Volz T, Allweiss L, Ben MM, et al. The entry inhibitor Myrcludex-B efficiently blocks intrahepatic virus spreading in humanized mice previously infected with hepatitis B virus. J Hepatol 2013;58:861–7.

59. Watashi K, Urban S, Li W, et al. NTCP and beyond: opening the door to unveil hepatitis B virus entry. Int J Mol Sci 2014;15:2892–905.

60. Ni Y, Lempp FA, Mehrle S, et al. Hepatitis B and D viruses exploit sodium taurocholate co-transporting polypeptide for species-specific entry into hepatocytes. Gastroenterology 2014;146:1070–83.

61. Watashi K, Sluder A, Daito T, et al. Cyclosporin A and its analogs inhibit hepatitis B virus entry into cultured hepatocytes through targeting a membrane transporter, sodium taurocholate cotransporting polypeptide (NTCP). Hepatology 2014;59:1726–37.

62. Lin SR, Yang HC, Kuo YT, et al. The CRISPR/Cas9 system facilitates clearance of the intrahepatic HBV templates in vivo. Mol Ther Nucleic Acids 2014;3:e186.

63. Karimova M, Beschorner N, Dammermann W, et al. CRISPR/Cas9 nickase-mediated disruption of hepatitis B virus open reading frame S and X. Sci Rep 2015;5:13734.

64. Kennedy EM, Bassit LC, Mueller H, et al. Suppression of hepatitis B virus DNA accumulation in chronically infected cells using a bacterial CRISPR/Cas RNA-guided DNA endonuclease. Virology 2015;476:196–205.

65. Ramanan V, Shlomai A, Cox DB, et al. CRISPR/Cas9 cleavage of viral DNA efficiently suppresses hepatitis B virus. Sci Rep 2015;5:10833.

66. Turelli P, Mangeat B, Jost S, et al. Inhibition of hepatitis B virus replication by APOBEC3G. Science 2004;303:1829.

67. Rosler C, Kock J, Kann M, et al. APOBEC-mediated interference with hepadnavirus production. Hepatology 2005;42:301–9.

68. Baumert TF, Rosler C, Malim MH, et al. Hepatitis B virus DNA is subject to extensive editing by the human deaminase APOBEC3C. Hepatology 2007;46:682–9.

69. Lucifora J, Xia Y, Reisinger F, et al. Specific and nonhepatotoxic degradation of nuclear hepatitis B virus cccDNA. Science 2014;343:1221–8.

70. Wieland SF, Chisari FV. Stealth and cunning: hepatitis B and hepatitis C viruses. J Virol 2005;79:9369–80.

71. Wieland S, Thimme R, Purcell RH, et al. Genomic analysis of the host response to hepatitis B virus infection. Proc Natl Acad Sci U S A 2004;101:6669–74.

72. Dunn C, Peppa D, Khanna P, et al. Temporal analysis of early immune responses in patients with acute hepatitis B virus infection. Gastroenterology 2009;137: 1289–300.

73. Lok AS, Ghany MG, Watson G, et al. Predictive value of aminotransferase and hepatitis B virus DNA levels on response to interferon therapy for chronic hepatitis B. J Viral Hepat 1998;5:171–8.

74. Guidotti LG, Chisari FV. Immunobiology and pathogenesis of viral hepatitis. Annu Rev Pathol 2006;1:23–61.

75. Fisicaro P, Valdatta C, Boni C, et al. Early kinetics of innate and adaptive immune responses during hepatitis B virus infection. Gut 2009;58:974–82.

76. Hosel M, Quasdorff M, Wiegmann K, et al. Not interferon, but interleukin-6 controls early gene expression in hepatitis B virus infection. Hepatology 2009;50: 1773–82.

77. Guy CS, Mulrooney-Cousins PM, Churchill ND, et al. Intrahepatic expression of genes affiliated with innate and adaptive immune responses immediately after invasion and during acute infection with woodchuck hepadnavirus. J Virol 2008;82:8579–91.

78. Oliviero B, Varchetta S, Paudice E, et al. Natural killer cell functional dichotomy in chronic hepatitis B and chronic hepatitis C virus infections. Gastroenterology 2009;137:1151–60, 1160.e1–7.

79. Mondelli MU, Oliviero B, Mele D, et al. Natural killer cell functional dichotomy: a feature of chronic viral hepatitis? Front Immunol 2012;3:351.

80. Peppa D, Gill US, Reynolds G, et al. Up-regulation of a death receptor renders antiviral T cells susceptible to NK cell-mediated deletion. J Exp Med 2013;210: 99–114.

81. Lang PA, Contaldo C, Georgiev P, et al. Aggravation of viral hepatitis by platelet-derived serotonin. Nat Med 2008;14:756–61.

82. Guidotti LG, Inverso D, Sironi L, et al. Immunosurveillance of the liver by intravascular effector CD8(+) T cells. Cell 2015;161:486–500.

83. Martinet J, Dufeu-Duchesne T, Bruder Costa J, et al. Altered functions of plasmacytoid dendritic cells and reduced cytolytic activity of natural killer cells in patients with chronic HBV infection. Gastroenterology 2012;143:1586–96.e8.

84. Martinet J, Leroy V, Dufeu-Duchesne T, et al. Plasmacytoid dendritic cells induce efficient stimulation of antiviral immunity in the context of chronic hepatitis B virus infection. Hepatology 2012;56:1706–18.

85. Dunn C, Brunetto M, Reynolds G, et al. Cytokines induced during chronic hepatitis B virus infection promote a pathway for NK cell-mediated liver damage. J Exp Med 2007;204:667–80.

86. Pallett LJ, Gill US, Quaglia A, et al. Metabolic regulation of hepatitis B immunopathology by myeloid-derived suppressor cells. Nat Med 2015;21:591–600.

87. Tsutsumi Y, Yamamoto Y, Ito S, et al. Hepatitis B virus reactivation with a rituximab-containing regimen. World J Hepatol 2015;7:2344–51.

88. Rehermann B, Nascimbeni M. Immunology of hepatitis B virus and hepatitis C virus infection. Nat Rev Immunol 2005;5:215–29.

89. Das A, Ellis G, Pallant C, et al. IL-10-producing regulatory B cells in the pathogenesis of chronic hepatitis B virus infection. J Immunol 2012;189:3925–35.

90. Miller DJ, Dwyer JM, Klatskin G. Identification of lymphocytes in percutaneous liver biopsy cores. Different T: B cell ratio in HB sAg-positive and -negative hepatitis. Gastroenterology 1977;72(6):1199–203.

91. Ferrari C, Penna A, Bertoletti A, et al. Cellular immune response to hepatitis B virus-encoded antigens in acute and chronic hepatitis B virus infection. J Immunol 1990;145:3442–9.

92. Bertoletti A, Ferrari C, Fiaccadori F, et al. HLA class I-restricted human cytotoxic T cells recognize endogenously synthesized hepatitis B virus nucleocapsid antigen. Proc Natl Acad Sci U S A 1991;88:10445–9.

93. Jung MC, Stemler M, Weimer T, et al. Immune response of peripheral blood mononuclear cells to HBx-antigen of hepatitis B virus. Hepatology 1991;13: 637–43.

94. Penna A, Chisari FV, Bertoletti A, et al. Cytotoxic T lymphocytes recognize an HLA-A2-restricted epitope within the hepatitis B virus nucleocapsid antigen. J Exp Med 1991;174:1565–70.

95. Missale G, Redeker A, Person J, et al. HLA-A31- and HLA-Aw68-restricted cytotoxic T cell responses to a single hepatitis B virus nucleocapsid epitope during acute viral hepatitis. J Exp Med 1993;177:751–62.

96. Maini MK, Boni C, Ogg GS, et al. Direct ex vivo analysis of hepatitis B virus-specific CD8(+) T cells associated with the control of infection. Gastroenterology 1999;117:1386–96.

97. Thimme R, Wieland S, Steiger C, et al. CD8(+) T cells mediate viral clearance and disease pathogenesis during acute hepatitis B virus infection. J Virol 2003;77:68–76.

98. Xia Y, Stadler D, Lucifora J, et al. Interferon-gamma and tumor necrosis factor-alpha produced by T cells reduce the HBV persistence form, cccDNA, without cytolysis. Gastroenterology 2016;150:194–205.

99. Guidotti LG, Rochford R, Chung J, et al. Viral clearance without destruction of infected cells during acute HBV infection. Science 1999;284:825–9.

100. Boettler T, Panther E, Bengsch B, et al. Expression of the interleukin-7 receptor alpha chain (CD127) on virus-specific CD8+ T cells identifies functionally and phenotypically defined memory T cells during acute resolving hepatitis B virus infection. J Virol 2006;80:3532–40.

101. Maini MK, Boni C, Lee CK, et al. The role of virus-specific CD8(+) cells in liver damage and viral control during persistent hepatitis B virus infection. J Exp Med 2000;191:1269–80.

102. Zhang Z, Zhang JY, Wherry EJ, et al. Dynamic programmed death 1 expression by virus-specific CD8 T cells correlates with the outcome of acute hepatitis B. Gastroenterology 2008;134:1938–49, 1949.e1–3.

103. Kurktschiev PD, Raziorrouh B, Schraut W, et al. Dysfunctional CD8+ T cells in hepatitis B and C are characterized by a lack of antigen-specific T-bet induction. J Exp Med 2014;211:2047–59.

104. Boni C, Fisicaro P, Valdatta C, et al. Characterization of hepatitis B virus (HBV)-specific T-cell dysfunction in chronic HBV infection. J Virol 2007;81:4215–25.

105. Pauken KE, Wherry EJ. Overcoming T cell exhaustion in infection and cancer. Trends Immunol 2015;36:265–76.

106. Fisicaro P, Valdatta C, Massari M, et al. Antiviral intrahepatic T-cell responses can be restored by blocking programmed death-1 pathway in chronic hepatitis B. Gastroenterology 2010;138:682–93, 693.e1–4.

107. Fisicaro P, Valdatta C, Massari M, et al. Combined blockade of programmed death-1 and activation of CD137 increase responses of human liver T cells against HBV, but not HCV. Gastroenterology 2012;143:1576–85.e4.

108. Schurich A, Khanna P, Lopes AR, et al. Role of the coinhibitory receptor cytotoxic T lymphocyte antigen-4 on apoptosis-Prone CD8 T cells in persistent hepatitis B virus infection. Hepatology 2011;53:1494–503.

109. Nebbia G, Peppa D, Schurich A, et al. Upregulation of the Tim-3/galectin-9 pathway of T cell exhaustion in chronic hepatitis B virus infection. PLoS One 2012;7:e47648.

110. Cai G, Nie X, Li L, et al. B and T lymphocyte attenuator is highly expressed on intrahepatic T cells during chronic HBV infection and regulates their function. J Gastroenterol 2013;48:1362–72.

111. Bengsch B, Martin B, Thimme R. Restoration of HBV-specific CD8+ T cell function by PD-1 blockade in inactive carrier patients is linked to T cell differentiation. J Hepatol 2014;61:1212–9.

112. Knolle PA, Thimme R. Hepatic immune regulation and its involvement in viral hepatitis infection. Gastroenterology 2014;146:1193–207.

113. Iwai Y, Terawaki S, Ikegawa M, et al. PD-1 inhibits antiviral immunity at the effector phase in the liver. J Exp Med 2003;198:39–50.

114. El-Khoueiry A, Melero I, Crocenzi T, et al. Phase I/II safety and antitumor activity of nivolumab in patients with advanced hepatocellular carcinoma (HCC): CA209-040. J Clin Oncol 2015;33. Available at: http://meetinglibrary.asco.org/content/146146-156. Accessed July 22, 2016.

115. Raziorrouh B, Heeg M, Kurktschiev P, et al. Inhibitory phenotype of HBV-specific CD4+ T-cells is characterized by high PD-1 expression but absent coregulation of multiple inhibitory molecules. PLoS One 2014;9:e105703.

116. Park JJ, Wong DK, Wahed AS, et al. Hepatitis B virus-specific and global T-cell dysfunction in chronic hepatitis B. Gastroenterology 2016;150:684–95.e5.

117. Franzese O, Kennedy PT, Gehring AJ, et al. Modulation of the CD8+-T-cell response by CD4+ CD25+ regulatory T cells in patients with hepatitis B virus infection. J Virol 2005;79:3322–8.

118. Lopes AR, Kellam P, Das A, et al. Bim-mediated deletion of antigen-specific CD8 T cells in patients unable to control HBV infection. J Clin Invest 2008;118:1835–45.

119. Schurich A, Pallett LJ, Lubowiecki M, et al. The third signal cytokine IL-12 rescues the anti-viral function of exhausted HBV-specific CD8 T cells. PLoS Pathog 2013;9:e1003208.

120. Das A, Hoare M, Davies N, et al. Functional skewing of the global CD8 T cell population in chronic hepatitis B virus infection. J Exp Med 2008;205:2111–24.

121. Sandalova E, Laccabue D, Boni C, et al. Increased levels of arginase in patients with acute hepatitis B suppress antiviral T cells. Gastroenterology 2012;143:78–87.e3.

122. Rehermann B, Pasquinelli C, Mosier SM, et al. Hepatitis B virus (HBV) sequence variation of cytotoxic T lymphocyte epitopes is not common in patients with chronic HBV infection. J Clin Invest 1995;96:1527–34.

123. Dienstag JL, Stevens CE, Bhan AK, et al. Hepatitis B vaccine administered to chronic carriers of hepatitis b surface antigen. Ann Intern Med 1982;96:575–9.

124. Liang TJ, Block TM, McMahon BJ, et al. Present and future therapies of hepatitis B: from discovery to cure. Hepatology 2015;62:1893–908.
125. Heathcote J, McHutchison J, Lee S, et al. A pilot study of the CY-1899 T-cell vaccine in subjects chronically infected with hepatitis B virus. The CY1899 T Cell Vaccine Study Group. Hepatology 1999;30:531–6.
126. Yang SH, Lee CG, Park SH, et al. Correlation of antiviral T-cell responses with suppression of viral rebound in chronic hepatitis B carriers: a proof-of-concept study. Gene Ther 2006;13:1110–7.
127. Yoon SK, Seo YB, Im SJ, et al. Safety and immunogenicity of therapeutic DNA vaccine with antiviral drug in chronic HBV patients and its immunogenicity in mice. Liver Int 2015;35:805–15.
128. Gehring AJ, Haniffa M, Kennedy PT, et al. Mobilizing monocytes to cross-present circulating viral antigen in chronic infection. J Clin Invest 2013;123:3766–76.
129. June CH, Levine BL. T cell engineering as therapy for cancer and HIV: our synthetic future. Philos Trans R Soc Lond B Biol Sci 2015;370:20140374.
130. Krebs K, Bottinger N, Huang LR, et al. T cells expressing a chimeric antigen receptor that binds hepatitis B virus envelope proteins control virus replication in mice. Gastroenterology 2013;145:456–65.

Interferon Treatment for Hepatitis B

Monica A. Konerman, MD, MSc, Anna S. Lok, MD*

KEYWORDS

- Chronic hepatitis B • Cirrhosis • Hepatocellular carcinoma • Hepatitis B e antigen
- Hepatitis B surface antigen • Hepatitis B virus genotype

KEY POINTS

- Interferon (IFN) therapy offers several benefits over nucleos(t)ide analogs for treatment of chronic hepatitis B including a finite duration of therapy and a higher rate of clearance of hepatitis Be antigen and surface antigen.
- Patients who respond to IFN therapy have been shown to have improvement in clinical outcomes, specifically a decrease in incidence of hepatocellular carcinoma and development of cirrhosis.
- IFN is associated with a broad spectrum of potential adverse effects, including psychiatric effects, bone marrow suppression, and exacerbation of autoimmune diseases.
- Recommendations to use IFN should balance benefits versus risks and decisions should be tailored to individual patient characteristics and preference.

INTRODUCTION

Chronic hepatitis B virus (HBV) infection has a significant public health impact with roughly 250 million persons worldwide chronically infected.[1] HBV infection is a major cause of liver cirrhosis and is responsible for more than one-half of the cases of hepatocellular carcinoma (HCC) in the world. The course of chronic HBV infection is notable for fluctuations in viral replication and liver injury and disease progression is influenced by multiple host, virus, and environmental factors.

Currently, there are 7 approved therapies, including standard and pegylated (PEG) interferon (IFN)-α, and 5 nucleos(t)ide analogs (NUCs). The goal of therapy is to achieve sustained suppression of HBV replication, which in turn will prevent cirrhosis,

Dr A.S. Lok has received research grants and served as an advisor for Merck and Gilead; research grants from Bristol-Myers Squibb; and has served on the safety board for Glaxo Smith Kline. Dr M.A. Konerman has nothing to disclose.
Division of Gastroenterology, Department of Internal Medicine, University of Michigan Health System, 1500 East Medical Center Drive, Ann Arbor, MI 48109, USA
* Corresponding author. Division of Gastroenterology, University of Michigan Health System, 3912 Taubman Center, 1500 East Medical Center Drive, SPC 5362, Ann Arbor, MI 48109.
E-mail address: aslok@umich.edu

hepatic decompensation, and HCC. IFN-α was the first treatment approved for chronic HBV infection. Although it is associated with a wide range of adverse events and has to be administered parenterally, the strengths of IFN-α therapy include a finite duration of administration and a higher rate of clearance of hepatitis B e antigen (HBeAg) and hepatitis B surface antigen (HBsAg) compared with NUCs (**Table 1**). This article reviews the mechanisms of action, efficacy, and clinical use of IFN therapy for HBV infection.

MECHANISMS OF ACTION OF INTERFERON IN HEPATITIS B

IFNs have several therapeutic effects including antiviral, antiproliferative, and immunomodulatory. IFN-α, IFN-β, and IFN-γ have all been evaluated as treatment for hepatitis B. IFN-α is most well-studied and the only type of IFN approved for treatment of hepatitis B in most countries. The antiviral effects of IFN-α depend on its binding to specific receptors, which then triggers a series of intracellular events including activation of 2′,5′-oligoadenylate synthetase. IFN-α has been shown to inhibit HBV replication by decreasing the transcription of pregenomic RNA and subgenomic RNA. Recent studies showed that the effect of IFN-α on HBV transcription is partly mediated by epigenetic modifications of the HBV covalently closed circular DNA. It can also induce degradation of covalently closed circular DNA by induction of APOBEC3s, DNA editing enzymes that can degrade foreign but not host DNAs.[2,3] In addition to direct antiviral activity, IFN-α enhances cell-mediated immune response and clearance of infected hepatocytes (**Fig. 1**). The pleiotropic effects of IFN-α and its ability to repress/degrade covalently closed circular DNA account for the higher rate of durable response and loss of HBeAg and HBsAg compared with NUCs.

Table 1
Advantages and disadvantages of IFN versus NUC therapies for chronic hepatitis B

	IFN	NUCs	Advantage
Duration of treatment	Finite (approx. 12 mo)	Indefinite	IFN
Antiviral resistance	None	LMV > TBV > ADV > ETV/ TDF	IFN
HBeAg and HBsAg loss	Modest, Genotype Dependent	Rare	IFN
Route of administration	Injection	Oral	NUC
Antiviral activity	Modest	Potent: ETV/TDF/ TBV > LMV > ADV	NUC
Side effects	Common, Potentially Severe	Negligible	NUC
Safety in pregnancy	Pregnancy class C	Pregnancy class B: TBV and TDF Safety data in humans: LMV, TBV and TDF	NUC
Safety in decompensated cirrhosis or liver failure	No	Yes	NUC

Abbreviations: ADV, adefovir; ETV, entecavir; LMV, lamivudine; NUC, nucleos(t)ide analog; TBV, telbivudine; TDF, tenofovir.

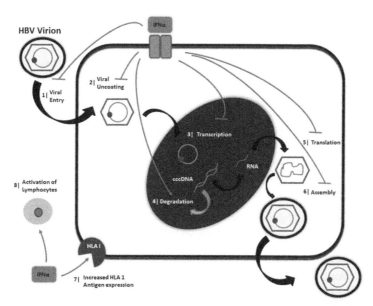

Fig. 1. Mechanism of action of interferon (IFN) therapy for chronic hepatitis B virus (HBV) infection. HBV lifecycle and mechanisms of action of IFN therapy in chronic hepatitis B. Potential effects of IFN include blocking (1) virus entry, (2) uncoating of virion, (3) transcription of viral DNA into RNA, (4) degradation of ccc DNA, (5) translation of viral RNA into proteins, (6) assembly of nucleocapsids, (7) increase HLA1 antigen expression, and (8) activation of CD8 T cells.

ENDPOINTS OF THERAPY

Response to antiviral therapy for CHB can be categorized as biochemical, serologic, virologic, or histologic.[4,5] It is further characterized as on-therapy or sustained off-therapy.[5] Responses to IFN occur slowly and HBeAg loss and HBsAg loss often continue to occur after completion of treatment. Thus, assessment of sustained off-therapy response is important in evaluating the benefits of IFN. Because alanine aminotransferase (ALT) flares are common during IFN treatment, assessment of biochemical and histologic responses is generally performed 6 months after completion of IFN treatment.[6,7] The ideal endpoint of CHB treatment is clearance of HBsAg with or without seroconversion to hepatitis B surface antibody. Although IFN is associated with a higher rate of HBsAg loss than NUCs, only 5% to 10% will clear HBsAg when assessed 24 weeks after completing a 1-year course of PEG IFN therapy. Thus, surrogate markers including normalization of ALT; suppression of serum HBV DNA levels to undetectable and loss of HBeAg with seroconversion to hepatitis B e antibody (anti-HBe) are usually used to evaluate response in clinical practice.

EFFICACY
Standard Interferon-α

Multiple studies have demonstrated the efficacy of standard IFN-α in CHB compared with no treatment, but it is rarely used in current practice.[8–10]

Hepatitis B e antigen positive
Several metaanalyses have confirmed a beneficial effect of standard IFN-α therapy in patients who are HBeAg positive. When response is assessed 6 to 12 months post

treatment, IFN-treated patients had higher rates of HBeAg loss (33% vs 12%), unde-tectable HBV DNA (37% vs 17%), and HBsAg loss (7.8% vs 1.8%) compared with un-treated controls.[10] The durability of HBeAg seroconversion is up to 90% and sustained suppression of HBV replication is usually accompanied by normalization of serum ALT levels and decrease in inflammation on biopsy.

Hepatitis B e antigen negative

Trials of standard IFN-α treatment in HBeAg-negative patients have shown decreases in HBV DNA and ALT levels,[8,9] but relapse after cessation of treatment is frequent, with sustained response rates of only 15% to 30%.[11–14] Some studies have advocated longer durations of therapy (24 months).[11,15]

Pegylated Interferon-α

Attachment of a polyethylene glycol molecule to IFN (pegylation) reduces the rate of absorption and renal and cellular clearance resulting in a longer half-life compared with standard IFN. PEG IFN requires less frequent dosing and has been shown in clin-ical trials to yield more sustained viral suppression compared with standard IFN.[16] Two formulations have been evaluated (PEG IFN-α-2a and PEG IFN-α-2b), although only the α-2a formulation is available in most parts of the world. Studies have demon-strated similar efficacy of these formulations (**Table 2**).

Hepatitis B e antigen positive

Approval of PEG IFN for patients with HBeAg-positive CHB was based on a random-ized controlled trial evaluating the efficacy of PEG IFN-α-2a monotherapy versus lam-ivudine (LMV) monotherapy versus combination therapy administered for 48 weeks.[17] Patients treated with PEG IFN monotherapy or combination therapy were significantly more likely to achieve endpoints of interest compared with those treated with LMV monotherapy when assessed 24 weeks after completion of treatment: HBeAg seroconversion (32% and 27% vs 19%), HBV DNA less than approximately 20,000 IU/mL (32% and 34% vs 22%), and HBsAg loss (3% vs 0%). Serious adverse events occurred in 4% and 6% versus 2% of patients, who received PEG IFN, com-bination therapy, and LMV, respectively.

Similar response rates have been demonstrated in other studies. A 1-year course of PEG IFN-α-2b resulted in HBeAg seroconversion in roughly 30% to 36% patients and HBV DNA level less than approximately 20,000 IU/mL in 32% when assessed 24 weeks after cessation of treatment.[17–21] Responses assessed at a mean of 3.0 ± 0.8 years after completion of treatment showed 37% had lost HBeAg and 11% had lost HBsAg and durability of HBeAg seroconversion in 81% to 86% of initial responders.[22] A smaller study where PEG IFN-α-2b was administered for 32 weeks and LMV for 52 or 104 weeks, found that 77% of initial responders to PEG IFN had sustained HBeAg seroconversion and the combined HBeAg seroconversion rate, including initial nonresponders, increased to 60% at 5 years.[23]

Hepatitis B e antigen negative

Approval of PEG IFN-α for patients with HBeAg-negative CHB was based on a ran-domized controlled trial evaluating the efficacy of PEG IFN-α-2a monotherapy versus LMV monotherapy versus combination therapy for 48 weeks.[20] Patients treated with PEG IFN monotherapy or combination therapy were significantly more likely to achieve endpoints of interest compared with those treated with LMV monotherapy when assessed at week 72 (see **Table 2**). When these endpoints were assessed 3 years after the end of treatment, patients treated with PEG IFN were significantly more likely to have HBV DNA levels of approximately 2000 IU/mL or less (28% and 25% vs 15%) and to clear HBsAg (8% vs 0%).[24]

Monotherapy Versus Combination Therapy

The potential advantages of combining PEG IFN with NUCs are additive or synergistic antiviral effects, and diminished or delayed antiviral drug resistance. Most combination therapies evaluated have not been shown to be superior to PEG IFN monotherapy in inducing a higher rate of sustained response, but earlier studies combined PEG IFN with LMV, which has a low barrier to drug resistance and only evaluated simultaneous start and stop of both drugs.

Simultaneous start

Combination therapy of PEG IFN with LMV has not been shown to result in a significantly higher rate of sustained virologic response compared with PEG IFN alone.[17–20,22,23,25,26] A recent study found that the addition of tenofovir to PEG IFN increased the rate of HBsAg loss, although the benefit was primarily observed in HBeAg-positive patients and those infected with HBV genotype A. In this study, patients were randomized to receive tenofovir plus PEG IFN for 48 weeks (A) versus tenofovir plus PEG IFN for 16 weeks followed by tenofovir only for 32 weeks (B) versus tenofovir monotherapy for 120 weeks (C) versus PEG IFN monotherapy for 48 weeks (D).[27] At 72 weeks, 9%, 2.8%, 0%, and 2.8% of patients in these 4 groups had HBsAg loss. A subanalysis of patients in group A showed that of the rate of HBsAg loss for HBeAg positive and HBeAg negative patients was 9.3% and 5.1%, respectively, and were 37.5% and 33.3%, 11.1% and 8.7%, 5.3% and 4.8%, 6.7% and 0%, when stratified for HBV genotypes A, B, C, and D, respectively.

A small study evaluating a combination of PEG IFN and adefovir showed promising results, but this regimen is not recommended because of the weak antiviral activity of adefovir.[28]

One randomized trial comparing combination of PEG IFN and telbivudine versus monotherapy with either drug was terminated early owing to an increased incidence of peripheral neuropathy in the combination group.[29]

Add on or switch

Multiple studies have also evaluated the efficacy of sequential approaches with PEG IFN and NUCs. In 1 trial, HBeAg-positive Chinese patients were randomized to receive 48 weeks of PEG IFN alone or with 24 weeks of entecavir (either before or after initiation of PEG IFN).[30] HBeAg seroconversion assessed 24 weeks after treatment was not different in the 3 groups. A second trial randomized HBeAg-positive patients receiving entecavir to either continued entecavir monotherapy or add-on PEG IFN from weeks 24 to 48.[31] No significant benefit was noted when HBeAg loss and HBV DNA levels were assessed at weeks 48 or 96. A third study randomized HBeAg-positive patients who had been receiving entecavir for 9 to 36 months to continue entecavir monotherapy or to switch to PEG IFN for 48 weeks.[32] At week 48, patients switched to PEG IFN had a higher rate of HBeAg seroconversion than those on entecavir monotherapy but all patients in this study had low HBeAg titers at entry.

Subgroups

Lamivudine resistance

The efficacy of PEG IFN in patients with LMV resistance has not been extensively evaluated. In 1 study, HBeAg-positive patients were randomized to PEG IFN for 48 weeks (n = 155) or adefovir for 72 weeks (n = 80). At 6 months after treatment, those treated with PEG IFN had a significantly higher rate of HBeAg seroconversion (15% vs 4%).[33]

Table 2
Efficacy of PEG-IFN in chronic hepatitis B[a]

Study	n	Treatment Regimen	Duration (wk)	Response Timepoint	Definition of Sustained Response	Efficacy (%)
HBeAg positive						
Varying dose and duration						
Liaw et al,[19] 2011	544	1. PEG-IFNα-2a 90 μg/wk 2. PEG-IFNα-2a 90 μg/wk 3. PEG-IFNα-2a 180 μg/wk 4. PEG-IFNα-2a 180 μg/wk	24 48 24 48	24 wk post	HBeAg seroconversion HBV DNA <2000 IU/mL HBsAg loss	(1) 14, (2) 23, (3) 26, (4) 36 (1) 11, (2) 11, (3) 22, (4) 30 (1) 1, (2) 0, (3) 2, (4) 2
Simultaneous start						
Lau et al,[17] 2005	814	1. PEG-IFNα-2a 180 μg/wk + placebo 2. PEG-IFN, IFNα-2a 180 μg/wk + LMV 100 mg/d 3. LMV 100 mg/d	48	24 wk post	HBeAg seroconversion HBV DNA <100,000 copies/mL HBsAg loss	(1) 32, (2) 27, (3) 19 (1) 32, (2) 34, (3) 22 (1 +2) 3, (3) 0
Janssen et al,[26] 2005	307	1. PEG-IFNα-2b 100 μg/wk[b] + LMV 100 mg/d 2. PEG-IFN, IFNα-2b 100 μg/wk[b] + placebo	52	26 wk post	HBeAg loss	(1) 35%, (2) 36%
Buster et al,[22] 2008[c]	172		—	3 ± 0.8 y post	HBeAg loss HBV DNA <400 copies/mL HBsAg loss	(1) 36, (2) 37 (1) 13, (2) 26 (1) 15, (2) 8
Marcellin et al,[27] 2016	428	1. PEG-IFNα-2a 180 μg/wk + TDF × 48 wk 2. PEG-IFNα-2a 180 μg/wk +TDF × 16w -> TDF ×32 wk 3. TDF ×120w 4. PEG-IFNα-2a 180 μg/wk × 48 wk	48-120	24 wk post[d]	HBsAg loss HBeAg seroconversion	(1) 9, (2) 3, (3) 0, (4) 4 (1) 25, (2) 24, (3) 15, (4) 25
Switch						
Ning et al,[32] 2014	200	ETV for 9-36 m followed by: 1. PEG-IFNα-2a 180 μg/wk 2. ETV 0.5 mg/d	48	48 wk	HBeAg seroconversion HBsAg loss	(1) 15, (2) 6 (1) 8, (2) 0

Add on

Study	N	Treatment	Duration (wk)	Timepoint	Endpoint	Results
Chan et al,[18] 2005	100	1. PEG-IFNα-2b 1.5 μg/kg/w × 32 wk + LMV 52w 2. LMV 100 mg/d	52	24 wk post	HBeAg seroconversion and HBV DNA <500,0000 copies/mL	(1) 36, (2) 14
Xie et al,[30] 2014	218	1. PEG-IFNα-2b 100 μg/wk × 48 wk 2. PEG-IFNα-2b 100 μg/wk × 48 wk + ETV 0.5 mg/d wk 13–37 3. ETV × 24 wk + PEG-IFNα-2b 100 μg/wk, wk 21–48	48	24 wk post	HBeAg seroconversion	(1) 31, (2) 25, (3) 26
Brouwer et al,[31] 2015	175	1. ETV 0.5 mg/d 2. ETV 0.5 mg/d + PEG-IFNα 180 μg/wk, wk 24–48	48	48 wk post	HBeAg seroconversion	(1) 26, (2) 13

HBeAg negative

Simultaneous start

Study	N	Treatment	Duration (wk)	Timepoint	Endpoint	Results
Marcellin et al,[20,24] 2004/2009	537 315	1. PEG-IFNα-2a 180 μg/wk + placebo 2. PEG-IFNα-2a 180 μg/wk + LMV 100 mg/d 3. LMV 100 mg/d	48	24 wk post 3 y post	HBV DNA <400 copies/mL HBsAg loss HBV DNA ≤10,000 copies/mL HBsAg loss	(1) 19, (2) 20, (3) 7 (1 +2) 3, (3) 0 (1 +2) 28, (3) 15 (1 +2) 9, (3) 0
Marcellin et al,[27] 2016	312	1. PEG-IFNα-2a 180 μg/wk + TDF × 48 wk 2. PEG-IFNα-2a 180 μg/wk + TDF × 16 kw - > TDF ×32 wk 3. TDF ×120 wk 4. PEG-IFNα-2a 180 μg/wk × 48 wk	48-120	24 wk post[d]	HBsAg loss	(1) 5, (2) 1, (3) 0, (4) 1

Abbreviations: ETV, entecavir; HBeAg, hepatitis e antigen; HBsAg, hepatitis B surface antigen; HBV, hepatitis B virus; LMV, lamivudine; PEG-IFN, pegylated interferon; TDF, tenofovir.

[a] Includes only studies with n ≥100.
[b] Dose reduced to PEG-IFN 50 μg weekly (week 32–52).
[c] Represents a follow-up study of the above Janssen 2005 trial.
[d] For patients in group 3, endpoint was week 72 of treatment.

Although these data suggest that PEG IFN may be effective in some patients with LMV resistance, treatment with a different NUC that does not have cross-resistance, such as tenofovir, produces more consistent response and is the preferred treatment.[34,35]

Children

IFN has been shown to be effective in suppressing HBV replication and in inducing HBeAg loss in HBeAg-positive children with an elevated ALT.[7,36] A multinational randomized trial showed that 26% of treated children became HBeAg negative with undetectable HBV DNA at the end of 24 weeks of treatment as compared with 11% who were untreated.[37] PEG IFN has not been approved for use in the United States in the pediatric population.[36] It has been recommended for use in other countries, however.[38]

Pregnancy

IFN treatment is contraindicated during pregnancy.[7] A trial of PEG-IFN in women contemplating pregnancy in the future may be considered because the duration of treatment is only 1 year. Women of childbearing age who are considering IFN therapy should be counseled about the importance of contraception and pregnancy test should be performed before and during the course of therapy. If a patient becomes pregnant while on therapy, IFN should be stopped immediately.

Cirrhosis, severe hepatitis, or acute liver failure

As detailed elsewhere in this paper, IFN should be used with caution in patients with compensated cirrhosis. It is contraindicated in patients with decompensated cirrhosis, severe hepatitis, or acute liver failure.[7]

Impact on Clinical Outcomes

Results in terms of impact on clinical outcomes for patients treated with standard IFN are conflicting, but most studies demonstrate better overall survival and a decrease in the development of cirrhosis and some studies a reduced incidence of HCC as well.[39–42] In a study comparing 233 HBeAg-positive patients in Taiwan treated with IFN-α with matched controls over a median follow-up of 6.8 years, those who received IFN therapy had lower rates of progression to cirrhosis and among those with cirrhosis, patients receiving IFN were less likely to develop HCC.[41] Patients who are HBeAg negative and achieved a sustained response to IFN-α therapy may have improved clinical outcomes, including overall survival, hepatic decompensation, and HCC, although this benefit is not consistent across studies.[11,14] A recent metaanalysis evaluated 5 observational studies with a mean follow-up of 84 months and found that IFN-α therapy compared with no treatment significantly decreased the risk of HCC but not all-cause mortality or decompensated liver disease.[43–48]

Data regarding the impact of PEG-IFN therapy on clinical outcomes are limited. A recent retrospective study of 177 patients treated with NUCs and 153 patients treated with PEG IFN found a benefit of PEG IFN therapy in decreasing risk of HCC.[49]

Predictors of Response

Predictors of response to standard and PEG IFN-α are similar. Pretreatment predictors can help in selecting patients who are most likely to benefit from IFN treatment to initiate therapy and on-treatment predictors can help in identifying patients who are unlikely to respond such that treatment can be stopped and patients spared the unnecessary adverse events and costs.

Pretreatment factors

Various host, disease, and virus factors have been demonstrated to be associated with response in HBeAg-positive patients, but factors predictive of response in HBeAg-negative patients have not been shown consistently.

Host factors Female sex has been associated with a higher likelihood of response to IFN in some but not all studies.[50] Asian patients were shown in early studies of standard IFN to have lower response rates as compared with Caucasian patients, but this was largely related to the inclusion of patients with normal ALT.[51] Subsequent studies showed that HBeAg-positive patients with elevated ALT respond similarly to Caucasian patients.[51,52] Patients with a prior history of IFN therapy have lower response rates to retreatment with IFN.[50]

Disease factors High pretreatment ALT level ($>2\times$ the upper limit of normal [ULN]) has been shown to be the strongest predictor of favorable response in HBeAg-positive patients. A study of 79 Chinese patients demonstrated that sustained response to IFN-α was seen in 38% of patients with elevated pretreatment ALT compared with 5% of patients with normal pretreatment ALT.[51] A second study of 542 HBeAg-positive patients treated with PEG IFN had similar findings with abnormal ALT having an odds of 1.31 (95% confidence interval, 1.02–1.69) for response.[50] Patients with high histologic activity index also have higher rates of IFN-related HBeAg seroconversion. A high baseline ALT and histologic activity index likely reflect stronger pretreatment immune response to HBV.

Virus factors HBV genotype has been shown to be a predictor of response to IFN but not to NUC therapy. Among HBeAg-positive patients, genotype A infection is associated with a higher rate of loss of HBeAg and HBsAg.[26,50,53] Studies in Asia also showed that genotype B is associated with a higher rate of HBeAg loss than genotype C. Similar findings have been demonstrated among HBeAg negative patients, with higher response rates in patients with genotype A (59%) versus genotype D (29%).[54–56]

The presence of precore and core promoter variants has been reported to be associated with response to IFN treatment, although the finding is inconsistent across studies.[8,57,58]

Low pretreatment HBV DNA level has been found to be a positive predictor of response to IFN therapy.[50] A pooled analysis of 721 patients found that a model including age, sex, HBV genotype, ALT level, HBV DNA level, and prior IFN therapy predicted sustained response. The likelihood of sustained response was highest (54%) in patients with genotype A, baseline ALT 2 or more times the ULN, and pretreatment HBV DNA less than 9 $\log_{10}$ copies/mL and lowest (7%) in patients with genotype D, baseline ALT less than 2 times the ULN and HBV DNA of 9 log or greater.[50]

Low pretreatment HBsAg level has also been associated with a higher likelihood of response to PEG IFN therapy for both HBeAg-positive and HBeAg-negative patients, but predictive accuracy is lower than on-treatment changes in HBsAg level.[59,60]

On-treatment factors

Disease factors On-treatment elevations in ALT have been shown to be a predictor of response in both HBeAg-positive and in HBeAg-negative patients.[20] IFN therapy is associated with flares of ALT (generally defined as 3-fold increase) in 30% to 50% of HBeAg-positive patients and is thought to reflect immune-mediated lysis of infected hepatocytes.[6] The timing of ALT flare in relation to change in HBV DNA level seems to be important with "host-induced" flares (defined as an ALT flare followed by a decrease in HBV DNA level) being associated with HBeAg loss, whereas "virus induced" flares (defined as ALT flare occurring after an increase in HBV DNA level) not having this association.[61] Frequency of flares in HBeAg-negative patients during a 48- to 52-week course of PEG IFN therapy varied from 12% to 22% depending on the definition of flare.[20,62]

Virus factors Patients who go on to achieve a sustained viral response have more rapid decrease in HBV DNA levels, but on-treatment HBV DNA level is not a reliable predictor of sustained response.[50,60,63] Quantitative HBsAg is the strongest on-treatment factor in predicting likelihood of response to IFN therapy. Lack of or insufficient decline in HBsAg level after 12 weeks of PEG IFN therapy had been shown to have greater than 90% negative predictive value for sustained response.[64] Quantitative HBeAg had also been shown to correlate with response to PEG IFN therapy, but assays for HBeAg level are not widely available and the predictive accuracy has not been validated.[63,65–67]

Response-Guided Stop Rules

A decrease in the HBsAg level after 12 weeks of PEG IFN has been proposed as a stop rule to prevent futile treatment and to avoid unnecessary adverse events. Applying the stop rule will also maximize the cost effectiveness of PEG IFN therapy. However, the clinical usefulness of these rules has been limited owing to lack of prospective validation and requirement of different rules based on HBV genotype and HBeAg status (**Table 3**).[68]

CLINICAL USE
Patient Selection

The decision of whether to start or to defer treatment of CHB should balance the activity and stage of liver disease with the likelihood of success and potential risks of treatment. Patients with CHB and evidence of ongoing active viral replication (serum HBV DNA >20,000 IU/mL for HBeAg-positive and >2000 IU/mL for HBeAg-negative patients) and active liver disease (ALT >2× ULN or moderate to severe inflammation or fibrosis on liver biopsy) should receive treatment. PEG IFN, entecavir, and tenofovir are the preferred therapies (**Fig. 2**). Patients with genotype A infection, high pretreatment ALT, and low HBV DNA levels are most likely to respond and should be encouraged to try a course of PEG IFN first, particularly if they are not committed to long-term treatment.

Contraindications to Therapy

IFN is contraindicated in patients with decompensated cirrhosis given the risk of severe sepsis and worsening liver failure. IFN is also not recommended in patients with compensated cirrhosis and evidence of portal hypertension, in those with severe exacerbations of CHB, and in patients with acute liver failure. Patients with compensated cirrhosis and no clinical evidence of portal hypertension can be treated with IFN, but caution should be exercised because flares might lead to hepatic decompensation. Pregnant patients and patients who require antiviral prophylaxis while receiving immunosuppressive or cancer chemotherapy, patients with medical or psychiatric comorbidities that can be exacerbated by IFN, and those with baseline neutropenia or marked thrombocytopenia should not receive IFN.

Table 3
Quantitative HBsAg 12 week stop rule for IFN therapy in chronic hepatitis B

Study	n	Study Details	Stop Rule	Response Definition[a]	PPV (%)	NPV (%)
HBeAg Positive						
Sonneveld et al,[64] 2010	221	HBV 99-01 study PEG-IFNα-2b ± LMV for 52 wk	No decline in HBsAg	HBeAg loss and HBV DNA <10,000 copies/mL	25	97
Piratvisuth et al,[73] 2013	399	Phase 3 study PEG-IFNα-2a ± LMV for 48 wk	HBsAg <1500 IU/mL	HBeAg seroconversion	55	72
Liaw et al,[19] 2011	114	NEPTUNE study: PEG-IFNα-2a 180 μg/wk for 48 wk	1. HBsAg <1500 IU/mL 2. HBsAg >20,000 IU/mL	HBeAg seroconversion	1. 58 2. NR	1. 84 2. 100
Piratvisuth et al,[74] 2011	526	Combined analysis of phase III study PEG-IFNα-2a ± LMV and NEPTUNE study[b]	No decline in HBsAg	HBeAg loss and HBV DNA <10,000 copies/mL	NR	82 Phase III 71 NEPTUNE
Sonneveld et al,[75] 2013	779	Combined analysis of phase III study PEG-IFNα-2a ± LMV, NEPTUNE study[b], and HBV 99-01 study PEG-IFNα-2b ± LMV; With subanalysis of PEG-IFN monotherapy (n = 45)[a]	1. No decline in HBsAg for genotypes A and D 2. HBsAg >20,000 IU/mL for genotypes B and C	HBeAg loss and HBV DNA <2000 IU/mL	NR	1. 88-100 2. 92-98
HBeAg negative						
Marcellin et al,[76] 2008	160	Phase III study PEG-IFNα-2a ± LMV for 48 wk, subset with long-term follow-up data	HBsAg ≤1500 IU/mL	Clearance of HBsAg[c]	35	97
Moucari et al,[77] 2009	48	PEG-IFNα-2a for 48 wk	<0.5 log$_{10}$ decrease in HBsAg	Undetectable HBV DNA (<70 copies/mL)	89	90

(continued on next page)

Table 3
(continued)

Study	n	Study Details	Stop Rule	Response Definition[a]	PPV (%)	NPV (%)
Rijckborst et al,[78] 2012	160	Phase III study PEG-IFNα-2a ± LMV for 48 wk, subset with PEG-IFN monotherapy (n = 85) and PegBeLiver study PEG-IFNα-2a for 48–96 wk (n = 75)	No decline in HBsAg and <2 log HBV DNA decline	HBV DNA <2000 IU/mL and normal ALT	41	95
Peng et al,[79] 2012	61	PEG-IFNα-2a for 48 wk	HBsAg <150 IU/mL	Undetectable HBV DNA (<312 copies/mL)	86	85
Marcellin et al,[80] 2013	120	Phase III study PEG-IFN-α 2a ± LMV for 48 wk, subset with long-term follow-up data	≥10% $\log_{10}$ HBsAg decline	HBV DNA ≤2,000IU/mL[d]	42	87

Abbreviations: HBeAg, hepatitis B e antigen; HBsAg, hepatitis B surface antigen; HBV, hepatitis B virus; LMV, lamivudine; NEPTUNE, A Follow-up Study to Evaluate the Long-term Post Treatment Effects of Peginterferon Alfa-2a (PEG-IFN) in Patients With HBeAg Positive Chronic Hepatitis B From the Original Study WV19432; NPV, negative predictive value; NR, not reported; PEF-IFN, pegylated interferon; PPV, positive predictive value.

[a] Assessed at 6 months posttreatment unless otherwise indicated.
[b] Analysis limited to the group who received full dose (180 μg/week) PEG-IFN-α 2a for 48 weeks.
[c] Assessed at 4 years after end of treatment.
[d] Assessed at 5 years after end of treatment.

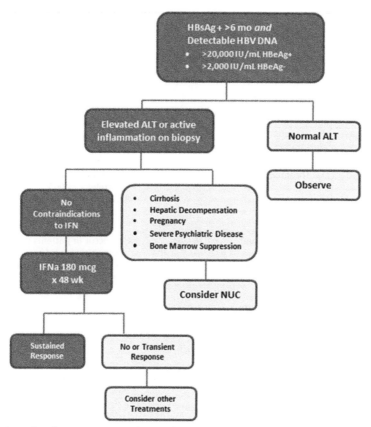

Fig. 2. Algorithm for treatment with interferon (IFN). ALT, alanine aminotransferase; HBV, hepatitis B virus; IFN, interferon; NUC, nucleos(t)ide analog.

Adverse Events

IFN therapy is associated with a wide range of adverse events that can be severe, limiting patient candidacy and often necessitate dose reductions or early termination of treatment (**Table 4**).[69] The most common side effect is an initial influenza-like illness. Other common side effects include fatigue, weight loss, anorexia, and emotional lability. The emotional side effects can be severe, resulting in suicidal ideation, and can occur in the absence of prior history of mental illness. As such, IFN should not be used in patients with active psychiatric disease or a history of suicidal tendency. Bone marrow suppression with a decrease in white cell and platelet counts is common and may necessitate dose reduction and in rare cases termination of treatment. Although neutropenia is a common adverse event, it is not correlated with an increased risk of infection.[70] IFN-α can induce the development of a variety of autoantibodies, although they are seldom accompanied by clinical sequelae with the exception of thyroid abnormalities. IFN-α can unmask or exacerbate autoimmune illnesses and should not be used in patients with underlying autoimmune diseases.

Dose Regimens

Both standard and PEG IFN are subcutaneously administered. Standard IFN-α is given in doses of 5 million units daily or 10 million units 3 times a week. For

Table 4
Adverse events associated with IFN therapy

System	Clinical Manifestations	Incidence (%)[a]	Details
Systemic	Flulike syndrome: fever, chills, myalgias, malaise, anorexia, headache	90	Typical onset 1–2 h after administration Symptoms usually dissipate within 24 h and diminish after first 1–2 injections
Hematologic	• Anemia • Leukopenia/ neutropenia • Thrombocytopenia	—	Typically seen within 1–3 wk of initiation of therapy Recovery within 3 wk of cessation Discontinue if ANC <500/mm³ or platelet <25,000 Neutropenia does not correlate with risk of infection in patients with compensated liver disease
Psychiatric	• Depression and anxiety • Emotional lability • Sleep disturbance	16–28	May occur in patients with no prior history and can be severe, including suicidal/homicidal ideation
Endocrine and metabolic	• Hyper/ hypothyroidism • Hyperglycemia • Hypertriglyceridemia	30 <5	
Gastrointestinal	• Diarrhea • Abdominal pain • Nausea and vomiting	20–30 12 33–39	
Hepatic	Increase in AST/ALT	12–50	May indicate augmented immune mediated clearance of infected hepatocytes and is a predictor of response, particularly if AST/ALT increase is followed by decline in serum HBV DNA IFN treatment can be continued in the absence of symptoms or increase in bilirubin level Severe flare can lead to hepatic decompensation and death
Dermatologic	• Injection site reactions • Alopecia	≤30 10–20	Discontinue for patients with acute hypersensitivity reaction

Abbreviations: ALT, alanine aminotransferase; ANC, absolute neutrophil count; AST, aspartate aminotransferase; IFN, interferon.
  [a] Listed when reported.

HBeAg-positive patients, 16 to 32 weeks of therapy are recommended.[71] HBeAg-negative patients require longer courses (1–2 years).[11] The recommended dose of PEG IFN-α-2a for both HBeAg-positive and HBeAg-negative patients is 180 μg weekly for 48 weeks. One trial comparing 180- versus 90-μg doses and 48 versus 24 weeks treatment in HBeAg-positive patients found that HBeAg seroconversion rate was highest in the group that received 180 μg doses for 48 weeks.[19] For HBeAg-negative patients, 1 study suggested that a 96-week course of PEG IFN may confer additional benefit compared with 48-week treatment.[72]

Table 5
Monitoring during IFN treatment

Parameter	Baseline	Week 4	Week 12	Week 24	Week 48	12 Weeks Post	24 Weeks Post	48 Weeks Post
CBC with differential	X	X	X	X	X	X	X	X
Hepatic panel	X	X	X	X	X	X	X	X
HBV DNA	X	—	X	X	X	X	X	X
HBeAg and anti-HBeAg[a]	X	—	—	X	X	X	X	X
HBsAg	X	—	—	—	X[b]	—	X[b]	X[b]
Quantitative HBsAg[c]	X	—	X	—	—	—	—	—
INR	X	—	—	—	—	—	—	—
TSH	X	—	X	X	X	X	—	—
Creatinine	X	—	—	—	—	—	—	—
Triglycerides	X	—	—	—	—	—	—	—
Glucose	X	—	—	—	—	—	—	—
Pregnancy test[d]	X	—	X	X	X	—	—	—

Abbreviations: CBC, complete blood count; HBeAg, hepatitis B e antigen; HBsAg, hepatitis B surface antigen; HBV, hepatitis B virus; IFN, interferon; INR, international normalized ratio; TSH, thyroid-stimulating hormone.
[a] For HBeAg-positive patients.
[b] For HBeAg-negative patients if HBV DNA is undetectable and for HBeAg-positive patients who have undergone HBeAg seroconversion.
[c] If Available to assess utility of continued therapy.
[d] For women of childbearing age.

Monitoring During Treatment

Patients receiving IFN therapy should be monitored closely during and after treatment. Both clinical assessment and laboratory testing are necessary to detect adverse events, and to evaluate response and appropriateness of continuing treatment. The recommended schedule of laboratory monitoring is outlined in **Table 5**.

SUMMARY

IFN therapy offers several benefits over NUCs for treatment of CHB, including a finite duration of therapy and a higher rate of clearance of HBeAg and HBsAg. Patients who respond to IFN therapy have been shown to have improvement in clinical outcomes. IFN is associated with a broad spectrum of potential adverse effects and recommendations to use IFN should balance benefits versus risks and decisions tailored to individual patient characteristics and preference.

REFERENCES

1. Ott JJ, Stevens GA, Groeger J, et al. Global epidemiology of hepatitis B virus infection: new estimates of age-specific HBsAg seroprevalence and endemicity. Vaccine 2012;30:2212–9.
2. Belloni L, Allweiss L, Guerrieri F, et al. IFN-alpha inhibits HBV transcription and replication in cell culture and in humanized mice by targeting the epigenetic regulation of the nuclear cccDNA minichromosome. J Clin Invest 2012;122:529–37.
3. Lucifora J, Xia Y, Reisinger F, et al. Specific and nonhepatotoxic degradation of nuclear hepatitis B virus cccDNA. Science 2014;343:1221–8.
4. European Association for the Study of the Liver. EASL clinical practice guidelines: management of chronic hepatitis B virus infection. J Hepatol 2012;57:167–85.
5. Lok AS, Heathcote EJ, Hoofnagle JH. Management of hepatitis B: 2000–summary of a workshop. Gastroenterology 2001;120:1828–53.
6. Nair S, Perrillo RP. Serum alanine aminotransferase flares during interferon treatment of chronic hepatitis B: is sustained clearance of HBV DNA dependent on levels of pretreatment viremia? Hepatology 2001;34:1021–6.
7. Terrault NA, Bzowej NH, Chang KM, et al. AASLD guidelines for treatment of chronic hepatitis B. Hepatology 2016;63:261–83.
8. Brunetto MR, Giarin M, Saracco G, et al. Hepatitis B virus unable to secrete e antigen and response to interferon in chronic hepatitis B. Gastroenterology 1993;105:845–50.
9. Fattovich G, Farci P, Rugge M, et al. A randomized controlled trial of lymphoblastoid interferon-alpha in patients with chronic hepatitis B lacking HBeAg. Hepatology 1992;15:584–9.
10. Wong DK, Cheung AM, O'Rourke K, et al. Effect of alpha-interferon treatment in patients with hepatitis B e antigen-positive chronic hepatitis B. A meta-analysis. Ann Intern Med 1993;119:312–23.
11. Lampertico P, Del Ninno E, Vigano M, et al. Long-term suppression of hepatitis B e antigen-negative chronic hepatitis B by 24-month interferon therapy. Hepatology 2003;37:756–63.
12. Luo K, Mao Q, Karayiannis P, et al. Tailored regimen of interferon alpha for HBeAg-positive chronic hepatitis B: a prospective controlled study. J Viral Hepat 2008;15:684–9.

13. Manesis EK, Hadziyannis SJ. Interferon alpha treatment and retreatment of hepatitis B e antigen-negative chronic hepatitis B. Gastroenterology 2001;121: 101–9.

14. Papatheodoridis GV, Manesis E, Hadziyannis SJ. The long-term outcome of interferon-alpha treated and untreated patients with HBeAg-negative chronic hepatitis B. J Hepatol 2001;34:306–13.

15. Lampertico P, Del Ninno E, Manzin A, et al. A randomized, controlled trial of a 24-month course of interferon alfa 2b in patients with chronic hepatitis B who had hepatitis B virus DNA without hepatitis B e antigen in serum. Hepatology 1997; 26:1621–5.

16. Cooksley WG, Piratvisuth T, Lee SD, et al. Peginterferon alpha-2a (40 kDa): an advance in the treatment of hepatitis B e antigen-positive chronic hepatitis B. J Viral Hepat 2003;10:298–305.

17. Lau GK, Piratvisuth T, Luo KX, et al. Peginterferon Alfa-2a, lamivudine, and the combination for HBeAg-positive chronic hepatitis B. N Engl J Med 2005;352: 2682–95.

18. Chan HL, Leung NW, Hui AY, et al. A randomized, controlled trial of combination therapy for chronic hepatitis B: comparing pegylated interferon-alpha2b and lamivudine with lamivudine alone. Ann Intern Med 2005;142:240–50.

19. Liaw YF, Jia JD, Chan HL, et al. Shorter durations and lower doses of peginterferon alfa-2a are associated with inferior hepatitis B e antigen seroconversion rates in hepatitis B virus genotypes B or C. Hepatology 2011; 54:1591–9.

20. Marcellin P, Lau GK, Bonino F, et al. Peginterferon alfa-2a alone, lamivudine alone, and the two in combination in patients with HBeAg-negative chronic hepatitis B. N Engl J Med 2004;351:1206–17.

21. Piratvisuth T, Lau G, Chao YC, et al. Sustained response to peginterferon alfa-2a (40 kD) with or without lamivudine in Asian patients with HBeAg-positive and HBeAg-negative chronic hepatitis B. Hepatol Int 2008;2:102–10.

22. Buster EH, Flink HJ, Cakaloglu Y, et al. Sustained HBeAg and HBsAg loss after long-term follow-up of HBeAg-positive patients treated with peginterferon alpha-2b. Gastroenterology 2008;135:459–67.

23. Wong VW, Wong GL, Yan KK, et al. Durability of peginterferon alfa-2b treatment at 5 years in patients with hepatitis B e antigen-positive chronic hepatitis B. Hepatology 2010;51:1945–53.

24. Marcellin P, Bonino F, Lau GK, et al. Sustained response of hepatitis B e antigen-negative patients 3 years after treatment with peginterferon alpha-2a. Gastroenterology 2009;136:2169–79.e1-4.

25. Brunetto MR, Oliveri F, Coco B, et al. Outcome of anti-HBe positive chronic hepatitis B in alpha-interferon treated and untreated patients: a long term cohort study. J Hepatol 2002;36:263–70.

26. Janssen HL, van Zonneveld M, Senturk H, et al. Pegylated interferon alfa-2b alone or in combination with lamivudine for HBeAg-positive chronic hepatitis B: a randomised trial. Lancet 2005;365:123–9.

27. Marcellin P, Ahn SH, Ma X, et al. Combination of tenofovir disoproxil fumarate and peginterferon alpha-2a increases loss of hepatitis B surface antigen in patients with chronic hepatitis B. Gastroenterology 2016;150:134–44.e110.

28. Lutgehetmann M, Volzt T, Quaas A, et al. Sequential combination therapy leads to biochemical and histological improvement despite low ongoing intrahepatic hepatitis B virus replication. Antivir Ther 2008;13:57–66.

29. Marcellin P, Wursthorn K, Wedemeyer H, et al. Telbivudine plus pegylated interferon alfa-2a in a randomized study in chronic hepatitis B is associated with an unexpected high rate of peripheral neuropathy. J Hepatol 2015;62:41–7.
30. Xie Q, Zhou H, Bai X, et al. A randomized, open-label clinical study of combined pegylated interferon Alfa-2a (40KD) and entecavir treatment for hepatitis B "e" antigen-positive chronic hepatitis B. Clin Infect Dis 2014;59:1714–23.
31. Brouwer WP, Xie Q, Sonneveld MJ, et al. Adding pegylated interferon to entecavir for hepatitis B e antigen-positive chronic hepatitis B: a multicenter randomized trial (ARES study). Hepatology 2015;61:1512–22.
32. Ning Q, Han M, Sun Y, et al. Switching from entecavir to PegIFN alfa-2a in patients with HBeAg-positive chronic hepatitis B: a randomised open-label trial (OSST trial). J Hepatol 2014;61:777–84.
33. Sun J, Hou JL, Xie Q, et al. Randomised clinical trial: efficacy of peginterferon alfa-2a in HBeAg positive chronic hepatitis B patients with lamivudine resistance. Aliment Pharmacol Ther 2011;34:424–31.
34. Fung S, Kwan P, Fabri M, et al. Randomized comparison of tenofovir disoproxil fumarate vs emtricitabine and tenofovir disoproxil fumarate in patients with lamivudine-resistant chronic hepatitis B. Gastroenterology 2014;146:980–8.
35. van Bommel F, Wunsche T, Mauss S, et al. Comparison of adefovir and tenofovir in the treatment of lamivudine-resistant hepatitis B virus infection. Hepatology 2004;40:1421–5.
36. Jonas MM, Block JM, Haber BA, et al. Treatment of children with chronic hepatitis B virus infection in the United States: patient selection and therapeutic options. Hepatology 2010;52:2192–205.
37. Sokal EM, Conjeevaram HS, Roberts EA, et al. Interferon alfa therapy for chronic hepatitis B in children: a multinational randomized controlled trial. Gastroenterology 1998;114:988–95.
38. Lindh M, Uhnoo I, Blackberg J, et al. Treatment of chronic hepatitis B infection: an update of Swedish recommendations. Scand J Infect Dis 2008;40:436–50.
39. Lin SM, Sheen IS, Chien RN, et al. Long-term beneficial effect of interferon therapy in patients with chronic hepatitis B virus infection. Hepatology 1999;29:971–5.
40. Yuen MF, Hui CK, Cheng CC, et al. Long-term follow-up of interferon alfa treatment in Chinese patients with chronic hepatitis B infection: the effect on hepatitis B e antigen seroconversion and the development of cirrhosis-related complications. Hepatology 2001;34:139–45.
41. Lin SM, Yu ML, Lee CM, et al. Interferon therapy in HBeAg positive chronic hepatitis reduces progression to cirrhosis and hepatocellular carcinoma. J Hepatol 2007;46:45–52.
42. Piratvisuth T. Reviews for APASL guidelines: immunomodulator therapy of chronic hepatitis B. Hepatol Int 2008;2:140–6.
43. Lok AS, McMahon BJ, Brown RS Jr, et al. Antiviral therapy for chronic hepatitis B viral infection in adults: a systematic review and meta-analysis. Hepatology 2016;63:284–306.
44. Fattovich G, Giustina G, Realdi G, et al. Long-term outcome of hepatitis B e antigen-positive patients with compensated cirrhosis treated with interferon alfa. European Concerted Action on Viral Hepatitis (EUROHEP). Hepatology 1997;26:1338–42.
45. Mahmood S, Niiyama G, Kamei A, et al. Influence of viral load and genotype in the progression of Hepatitis B-associated liver cirrhosis to hepatocellular carcinoma. Liver Int 2005;25:220–5.

46. Benvegnu L, Chemello L, Noventa F, et al. Retrospective analysis of the effect of interferon therapy on the clinical outcome of patients with viral cirrhosis. Cancer 1998;83:901–9.

47. Ikeda K, Saitoh S, Suzuki Y, et al. Interferon decreases hepatocellular carcinogenesis in patients with cirrhosis caused by the hepatitis B virus: a pilot study. Cancer 1998;82:827–35.

48. Effect of interferon-alpha on progression of cirrhosis to hepatocellular carcinoma: a retrospective cohort study. International Interferon-alpha Hepatocellular Carcinoma Study Group. Lancet 1998;351:1535–9.

49. Liang KH, Hsu CW, Chang ML, et al. Peginterferon is superior to nucleos(t)ide analogues for prevention of hepatocellular carcinoma in chronic hepatitis B. J Infect Dis 2016;213(6):966–74.

50. Buster EH, Hansen BE, Lau GK, et al. Factors that predict response of patients with hepatitis B e antigen-positive chronic hepatitis B to peginterferon-alfa. Gastroenterology 2009;137:2002–9.

51. Lok AS, Wu PC, Lai CL, et al. A controlled trial of interferon with or without prednisone priming for chronic hepatitis B. Gastroenterology 1992;102:2091–7.

52. Marcellin P, Xie Q, Piratvisuth T, et al. 41 S-Collate COHORT 'REAL-LIFE' Study: efficacy and safety of peginterfERON alfa-2a (40KD) IN 1233 Patients with chronic hepatitis B according to whom it may concern: Asian and Caucasian race. J Hepatol 2013;58:S18.

53. Flink HJ, van Zonneveld M, Hansen BE, et al. Treatment with Peg-interferon alpha-2b for HBeAg-positive chronic hepatitis B: HBsAg loss is associated with HBV genotype. Am J Gastroenterol 2006;101:297–303.

54. Erhardt A, Blondin D, Hauck K, et al. Response to interferon alfa is hepatitis B virus genotype dependent: genotype A is more sensitive to interferon than genotype D. Gut 2005;54:1009–13.

55. Erhardt A, Ludwig AD, Brunetto M, et al. HBV genotypes are the strongest predictors of response to interferon-alfa treatment: multivariate evaluation in 1229 hepatitis B patients. Hepatology 2008;48:700A–1A.

56. Wiegand J, Hasenclever D, Tillmann HL. Should treatment of hepatitis B depend on hepatitis B virus genotypes? A hypothesis generated from an explorative analysis of published evidence. Antivir Ther 2008;13:211–20.

57. Sonneveld MJ, Rijckborst V, Zeuzem S, et al. Presence of precore and core promoter mutants limits the probability of response to peginterferon in hepatitis B e antigen-positive chronic hepatitis B. Hepatology 2012;56:67–75.

58. Yang HC, Chen CL, Shen YC, et al. Distinct evolution and predictive value of hepatitis B virus precore and basal core promoter mutations in interferon-induced hepatitis B e antigen seroconversion. Hepatology 2013;57:934–43.

59. Tangkijvanich P, Komolmit P, Mahachai V, et al. Low pretreatment serum HBsAg level and viral mutations as predictors of response to PEG-interferon alpha-2b therapy in chronic hepatitis B. J Clin Virol 2009;46:117–23.

60. Manesis EK, Hadziyannis ES, Angelopoulou OP, et al. Prediction of treatment-related HBsAg loss in HBeAG-negative chronic hepatitis B: a clue from serum HBsAg levels. Antivir Ther 2007;12:73–82.

61. Flink HJ, Sprengers D, Hansen BE, et al. Flares in chronic hepatitis B patients induced by the host or the virus? Relation to treatment response during Peg-interferon {alpha}-2b therapy. Gut 2005;54:1604–9.

62. Chang ML, Liaw YF. Hepatitis B flares in chronic hepatitis B: pathogenesis, natural course, and management. J Hepatol 2014;61:1407–17.

63. Tangkijvanich P, Komolmit P, Mahachai V, et al. Comparison between quantitative hepatitis B surface antigen, hepatitis B e-antigen and hepatitis B virus DNA levels for predicting virological response to pegylated interferon-alpha-2b therapy in hepatitis B e-antigen-positive chronic hepatitis B. Hepatol Res 2010;40:269–77.

64. Sonneveld MJ, Rijckborst V, Boucher CA, et al. Prediction of sustained response to peginterferon alfa-2b for hepatitis B e antigen-positive chronic hepatitis B using on-treatment hepatitis B surface antigen decline. Hepatology 2010;52:1251–7.

65. Chuaypen N, Posuwan N, Payungporn S, et al. Serum hepatitis B core-related antigen as a treatment predictor of pegylated interferon in patients with HBeAg-positive chronic hepatitis B. Liver Int 2016;36(6):827–36.

66. Sonneveld MJ, Rijckborst V, Cakaloglu Y, et al. Durable hepatitis B surface antigen decline in hepatitis B e antigen-positive chronic hepatitis B patients treated with pegylated interferon-alpha2b: relation to response and HBV genotype. Antivir Ther 2012;17:9–17.

67. Fried MW, Piratvisuth T, Lau GK, et al. HBeAg and hepatitis B virus DNA as outcome predictors during therapy with peginterferon alfa-2a for HBeAg-positive chronic hepatitis B. Hepatology 2008;47:428–34.

68. Konerman MA, Lok AS. Is it more cost-effective for patients with chronic hepatitis b to have a trial of interferon before considering nucleos(t)ide analogue therapy? Clin Gastroenterol Hepatol 2015;13:386–9.

69. Fried MW. Side effects of therapy of hepatitis C and their management. Hepatology 2002;36:S237–44.

70. Cooper CL, Al-Bedwawi S, Lee C, et al. Rate of infectious complications during interferon-based therapy for hepatitis C is not related to neutropenia. Clin Infect Dis 2006;42:1674–8.

71. Janssen HL, Gerken G, Carreno V, et al. Interferon alfa for chronic hepatitis B infection: increased efficacy of prolonged treatment. The European Concerted Action on Viral Hepatitis (EUROHEP). Hepatology 1999;30:238–43.

72. Lampertico P, Vigano M, Di Costanzo GG, et al. Randomised study comparing 48 and 96 weeks peginterferon alpha-2a therapy in genotype D HBeAg-negative chronic hepatitis B. Gut 2013;62:290–8.

73. Piratvisuth T, Marcellin P, Popescu M, et al. Hepatitis B surface antigen: association with sustained response to peginterferon alfa-2a in hepatitis B e antigen-positive patients. Hepatol Int 2013;7(2):429–36.

74. Piratvisuth T, Marcellin P. Further analysis is required to identify an early stopping rule for peginterferon therapy that is valid for all hepatitis B e antigen-positive patients. Hepatology 2011;53:1054–5 [author reply: 1055].

75. Sonneveld MJ, Hansen BE, Piratvisuth T, et al. Response-guided peginterferon therapy in hepatitis B e antigen-positive chronic hepatitis B using serum hepatitis B surface antigen levels. Hepatology 2013;58:872–80.

76. Marcellin P, Brunetto M, Bonino F, et al. In patients with HBeAg-negative chronic hepatitis B HBsAg serum levels early during treatment with peginterferon alfa-2a predict HBsAg clearance 4 years post-treatment. Hepatology 2008;48:718A.

77. Moucari R, Mackiewicz V, Lada O, et al. Early serum HBsAg drop: a strong predictor of sustained virological response to pegylated interferon alfa-2a in HBeAg-negative patients. Hepatology 2009;49:1151–7.

78. Rijckborst V, Hansen BE, Ferenci P, et al. Validation of a stopping rule at week 12 using HBsAg and HBV DNA for HBeAg-negative patients treated with peginterferon alfa-2a. J Hepatol 2012;56:1006–11.

79. Peng CY, Lai HC, Li YF, et al. Early serum HBsAg level as a strong predictor of sustained response to peginterferon alfa-2a in HBeAg-negative chronic hepatitis B. Aliment Pharmacol Ther 2012;35:458–68.
80. Marcellin P, Bonino F, Yurdaydin C, et al. Hepatitis B surface antigen levels: association with 5-year response to peginterferon alfa-2a in hepatitis B e-antigen-negative patients. Hepatol Int 2013;7:88–97.

Liver Fibrosis Reversion After Suppression of Hepatitis B Virus

Don C. Rockey, MD

KEYWORDS

- Cirrhosis • Regression • Viral suppression • Hepatocellular carcinoma • HIV
- Portal hypertension • Stellate cell

KEY POINTS

- Robust data indicate that fibrosis regresses in patients with advanced fibrosis and even histologic evidence of cirrhosis, after hepatitis B virus (HBV) viral suppression.
- Overall outcomes are improved in patients with HBV viral suppression, including in those with cirrhosis and complications of cirrhosis.
- The preferred agents in patients with cirrhosis are entecavir and tenofovir, primarily because the risk of breakthrough is low.
- The risk of subsequent development of hepatocellular carcinoma is reduced after viral suppression.
- Despite viral suppression, there seems to be some risk of complications such as portal hypertension and/or hepatocellular carcinoma, the latter most commonly in patients with cirrhosis.

INTRODUCTION

Hepatitis B virus (HBV) infection causes a huge burden of disease worldwide. With the advent of ever-expanding and highly effective compounds that suppress or even eradicate this virus, great strides have been made.

HBV infection is complicated in many regards, not only by the complexities of the virus and hepatocyte interaction, but also by the host immune response. It typically causes chronic inflammation, the precursor to hepatic fibrogenesis.[1] In the liver, ongoing fibrogenesis ultimately leads to cirrhosis. HBV cirrhosis affects millions of patients worldwide and is responsible for an extremely high burden of disease.[2]

Treatment of patients with HBV with nucleos(t)ide analogs is well-known to lead to rapid suppression of HBV replication with a concomitant reduction in inflammation.

Funding support: The author receives support from NIH grant (R01 DK098819).
Department of Internal Medicine, The Medical University of South Carolina, 96 Jonathan Lucas Street, 803 CSB, Charleston, SC 29425, USA
E-mail address: rockey@musc.edu

Further, this suppression of inflammation provides an intrahepatic milieu such that fibrosis reverses, and further, an improvement in liver function and even survival in patients with complications of cirrhosis. In fact, the data in this area are overwhelmingly positive.

REVERSIBILITY OF FIBROSIS AND CIRRHOSIS

There is now extensive evidence that liver fibrosis regresses, both in experimental models[3] and in human liver disease (for the purposes of this discussion, it is assumed that reversion of fibrosis occurs along a continuum, whether linear or not, and that reversion of fibrosis and reversal of fibrosis may be partial or even complete). These data are highly consistent with the idea that liver wounding, as well as that in essentially all parenchymal organs, is a dynamic process that includes both matrix synthesis and deposition and matrix degradation.[1,4]

Further, the data also suggest that fibrosis and even cirrhosis regression is characteristic of virtually all forms of liver disease, and occurs in both experimental models[3,5,6] and in human liver disease[7-14] (**Fig. 1**). Currently available data suggest that, for fibrosis to regress, the underlying disease must be treated, either held in check or cured. This is especially true for liver diseases in which inflammation drives the fibrotic response (see below). Consistent with this concept are data in the HBV field in which there is fairly extensive evidence.[10,15-18] Active HBV typically drives inflammation and aggressive fibrogenesis, and elimination of this inflammatory response is associated with a reduction in fibrosis. Further, data are also now emerging in patients with hepatitis C virus infection.[19-21] Further, evidence exists in many other liver diseases as well, including delta hepatitis,[22] hemochromatosis,[23,24] removal of alcohol in alcoholic liver disease,[25] decompression of biliary obstruction in chronic pancreatitis,[12] immunosuppressive treatment of autoimmune liver disease,[14] and schistosomiasis.[26]

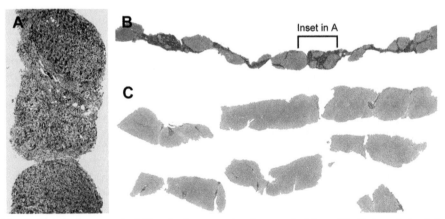

Fig. 1. Histologic reversal of fibrosis. An example of reversal of hepatitis B virus cirrhosis is shown. In (A) and (B) is shown liver histology from a biopsy before lamivudine treatment. In (C), after treatment with lamivudine, liver biopsy was repeated, and liver histology reveals almost complete dissolution of fibrosis. Similar data have been found in patients with autoimmune liver disease, alcoholic hepatitis, hepatitis C, and others. (*From* Wanless IR, Nakashima E, Sherman M. Regression of human cirrhosis. Morphologic features and the genesis of incomplete septal cirrhosis. Arch Pathol Lab Med 2000;124:1599–607; with permission.)

BASIC MECHANISMS

The pathogenesis of all forms of fibrosis is linked to a population of effector cells that produce abnormal amounts of extracellular matrix that is deposited in parenchymal tissue and disrupts organ function.[1] Further, implicit in this biology is that fibrosis is dynamic, and that there is not only deposition of extracellular matrix, but also that there is also resorption of this matrix. When imbalanced, the result is exaggerated fibrosis, or reversion of fibrosis (**Fig. 2**).

In the liver, the primary effector cell is the hepatic stellate cell (**Fig. 3**), which exhibits a number of key phenotypic characteristics during its activation that in turn drive the fibrogenic response.[4] In most forms of fibrogenesis, inflammation is a core driver of the fibrotic lesion (**Fig. 4**). This is particularly noteworthy in patients with HBV fibrosis and cirrhosis.

There are undoubtedly multiple mechanisms underlying fibrosis regression. A core concept is that during reversal of fibrosis, there seems to be a specific reduction in stellate cell activation (**Fig. 5**). Extensive data indicate that, in cell culture models, stellate cells can be manipulated such that they undergo a transition from an activated to a quiescent state.[27,28] This phenotypic reversal also occurs in vivo, although "deactivated" stellate cells seem to exhibit greater responsiveness to recurring fibrogenic stimulation.[29] Apoptosis of stellate cells also likely accounts for the decrease in number of activated stellate cells typical of resolution of hepatic fibrosis in vivo.[30] Apoptosis may be inhibited by factors present during injury, or stimulated by other

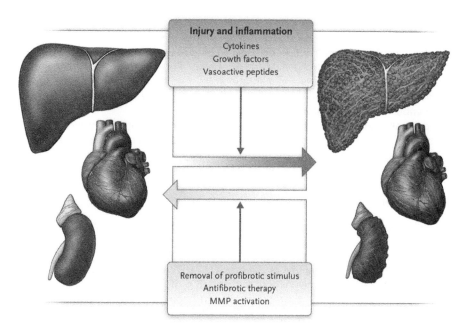

Fig. 2. Reversal of organ fibrosis. Fibrosis is remarkably plastic. In many, although not all instances, tissue fibrosis can be reversed as extracellular matrix proteins are degraded. Often, removal of the inciting stimulus is sufficient, and in a few instances, therapeutic interventions targeting the underlying disease process contribute as well. MMP, matrix metalloproteinase. (*From* Rockey DC, Bell PD, Hill JA. Fibrosis – a common pathway to organ injury and failure. N Engl J Med 2015;372:1145; with permission.)

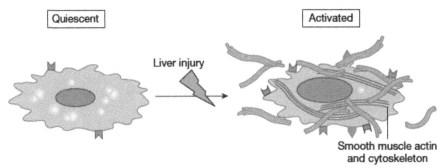

Quiescent   Activated

Liver injury

Smooth muscle actin
and cytoskeleton

Fig. 3. Stellate cell activation. A key pathogenic feature underlying liver fibrosis and cirrhosis is activation of hepatic stellate cells (note that activation of other effector cells is likely to parallel that of stellate cells). The activation process is complex, both in terms of the events that induce activation and the effects of activation. Multiple and varied stimuli participate in the induction and maintenance of activation, including but not limited to cytokines, peptides, and the extracellular matrix itself. Phenotypic features of activation include production of extracellular matrix, loss of retinoids, proliferation, upregulation of smooth muscle proteins, secretion of peptides and cytokines (with autocrine effects on stellate cells and paracrine effects on other cells such as leukocytes and malignant cells; see **Fig. 4**), and upregulation of various cytokine and peptide receptors. Additionally, evidence indicates that stellate cells exhibit several cell fates that are likely to play a critical role in fibrosis regression, highlighted at the bottom of the figure. (*From* Rockey DC. Hepatic fibrosis. In: Yamada's Textbook of Gastroenterology. West Sussex (United Kingdom): Wiley and Sons, Ltd; 2016. p. 2073; with permission.)

factors as the injury is removed. Additionally, molecules regulating matrix degradation seem to be closely linked to survival and apoptosis. For example, matrix metalloproteinase (MMP)2 activity correlated with apoptosis, and MMP2 may be stimulated by apoptosis.[31] Inhibition of MMP2 activity by TIMP-1 also blocks apoptosis in response to a number of apoptotic stimuli.[32]

Additionally, programmed cell death seems to be linked to autophagy, which seems to stimulate stellate cell activation, and may contribute to the fibrogenic cascade.[33–36] Cellular senescence has also been proposed to play a role in fibrosis resolution,[37–39] although the evidence for this in stellate cells is modest.

CLINICAL CONSIDERATIONS

The evidence that effective long-term treatment of patients with HBV and advanced liver fibrosis and even cirrhosis improves clinical outcomes is convincing. Several clinical considerations are noteworthy (**Box 1**). One of the more convincing studies established this concept.[10] In this trial of patients with HBV and advanced fibrosis (Ishak stage $\geq$4) who received lamivudine or placebo, 8% of patients receiving lamivudine and 18% of those receiving placebo developed hepatocellular carcinoma, spontaneous bacterial peritonitis, bleeding gastroesophageal varices, or had death related to liver disease ($P = .001$; **Fig. 6**).[10] Although fibrosis regression was not documented histologically, other data in the field suggest that the mechanism for the response was almost certainly fibrosis regression. A final point is that, for reversion of fibrosis or cirrhosis to be sustained, suppression of HBV replication (with normalization of alanine aminotransferase) is essential. A recurrent theme is that the beneficial effects of treatment are not found when there is breakthrough.

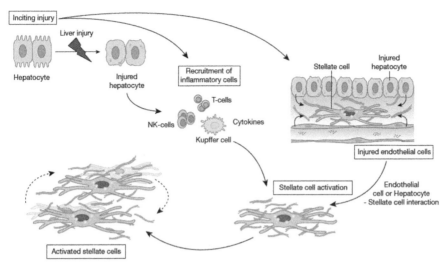

Fig. 4. The cellular response to wound healing. Most forms of liver injury result in hepatocyte injury, followed by inflammation, leading to activation of hepatic stellate cells. Inflammatory effectors are multiple and include T cells, natural killer (NK), and NK T cells, as well as Kupffer cells. These cells produce growth factors, cytokines, and chemokines that play an important role in stellate cell activation. Additionally, injury leads to disruption of the normal cellular environment, and also to stellate cell activation. Once activated, stellate cells themselves produce a variety of compounds, including growth factors, cytokines, chemokines, and vaso-active peptides. These substances have pleotrophic effects in the local environment, including autocrine effects on stellate cells themselves. Extracellular matrix synthesis, as well as production of matrix-degrading enzymes, are major consequences of stellate cell activation. (*From* Rockey DC. Hepatic fibrosis. In: Yamada's Textbook of Gastroenterology. West Sussex (United Kingdom): Wiley and Sons, Ltd; 2016. p. 2074; with permission.)

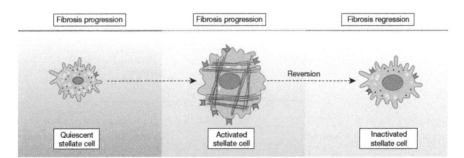

Fig. 5. The cellular mechanism of fibrosis reversion is linked to stellate cell phenotype. Activated hepatic stellate cells are removed from the fibrogenic milieu during fibrosis regression. The mechanism for their removal seems to be via their complete elimination (ie, via apoptosis) or via reversion from an activated to a quiescent phenotype. (*From* Rockey DC. Hepatic fibrosis. In: Yamada's Textbook of Gastroenterology. West Sussex (United Kingdom): Wiley and Sons, Ltd; 2016. p. 2077; with permission.)

Box 1
Critical issues associated with hepatitis B virus suppression/eradication

- How much fibrosis regression might be expected?
- Does it matter which antiviral agent is used?
- How long should the antiviral be used?
- How should fibrosis regression be measured?
- Does fibrosis reversion have an effect on clinical features of cirrhosis (such as quality of life, synthetic function, portal hypertension)?
- After viral suppression, what is the hepatocellular carcinoma risk?

Fibrosis Reversion After Hepatitis B Virus Suppression

Multiple agents with which to treat HBV are available currently. The evidence suggests that, so long as viral replication and the concomitant inflammatory response is suppressed, fibrosis will reverse. Thus, it probably does not matter so much which antiviral agent is used, but rather that it is important that the virus be suppressed or eliminated.

An important question to be addressed is exactly how much fibrosis regression should be expected. In one of the largest histologic studies of paired pretreatment and posttreatment liver biopsies[40] treated with an antiviral agent (in this study, tenofovir), 348 patients with HBV and advanced fibrosis had liver histology assessed at baseline and at 5 years (**Fig. 7**). In this group, viral suppression (HBV DNA <400 copies per mL) was documented in 330 of the 334 patients (99%) for whom viral load data were available. In the 96 patients (28%) with histologic cirrhosis (defined as Ishak score $\geq$5) at baseline, 71 (74%) had a reduction in fibrosis at year 5 (and thus did not have histologic cirrhosis). The difference between the proportion of patients with cirrhosis regression and without cirrhosis that progressed to cirrhosis (1%) was highly significant (*P*<.0001). Further, all but one with regression had a reduction of at least 2 units in the Ishak score at year 5, and more than one-half (58%, 56 patients) had a

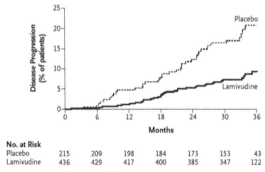

No. at Risk							
Placebo	215	209	198	184	173	153	43
Lamivudine	436	429	417	400	385	347	122

Fig. 6. Kaplan–Meier estimate of time to disease progression in patients with HBV treated with lamivudine. Patients were randomized to treatment with placebo or lamivudine, and followed for 36 months. Disease progression was defined as the development of hepatocellular carcinoma, spontaneous bacterial peritonitis, bleeding gastroesophageal varices, or had death related to liver disease. (*From* Liaw YF, Sung JJ, Chow WC, et al. Lamivudine for patients with chronic hepatitis B and advanced liver disease. N Engl J Med 2004;351:1521–31; with permission.)

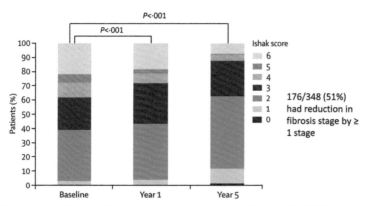

Fig. 7. Histology results over 5-year treatment phase in patients with HBV treated with tenofovir. The Ishak stage (0–6) of fibrosis in paired liver biopsy specimens from 348 patients at baseline, at 1 year, and at 5 years of treatment with tenofovir is shown (344 patients had specimens at all 3 time points). Of the 348 patients, 176 (51%) had reduction in fibrosis stage by 1 or more stages. (*From* Marcellin P, Gane E, Buti M, et al. Regression of cirrhosis during treatment with tenofovir disoproxil fumarate for chronic hepatitis B: a 5-year open-label follow-up study. Lancet 2013;381:468–75; with permission.)

decrease of 3 units or more. In the 252 patients (72%) who did not have histologic cirrhosis (Ishak score ≤4) at baseline, 12 (5%) had worse fibrosis at year 5; 135 (54%) had no change; and 105 (42%) had improvement. Nine of 12 patients with worsening had an increase in fibrosis score of 1 unit, and 3 patients (1%) progressed to cirrhosis.

In terms of the different HBV antiviral agents, they all seem to have substantial effectiveness in terms of their effects on reversion of advanced fibrosis (**Table 1**).[16,40–46] It should be emphasized that the general trends in terms of regression are remarkable, and that a majority of patients, but not all patients, should be expected to have fibrosis regression. Again, it is important to emphasize that this occurs in the setting of suppression of viral replication. Interestingly, it is unclear why some patients do not exhibit reversion of fibrosis, although it may be speculated that this has to do with host-specific fibrogenic factors.

In terms of the duration of treatment, the data suggest long-term therapy with antivirals is desirable. In the study (see **Fig. 7**)[40] of tenofovir, as discussed, this agent

Table 1
Effect of antiviral treatment on hepatitis B virus advanced fibrosis/cirrhosis reversion

Agent	N (Patients)	Fibrosis Reversion (%)	Time (y)	Ref
Lamivudine	30	67	3	41
	24	46	3	42
	47	49	1	45
Adefovir	12	58	5	43
	15	60	5	44
Entecavir	97	57–59	1	45
	13	85	3	46
	10	100	5	16
Tenofovir	96	74	5	17

seemed to be safe and effective when given for 5 years, and there is no reason to believe that even longer term treatment would not be safe. Further, given the natural history of HBV cirrhosis, it is expected that the longer the durability of viral suppression, the greater the effect on clinical outcomes.

Measurement of Fibrosis

Measurement of fibrosis is important for several reasons. First, it helps to stage liver disease, but also to monitor fibrosis after therapy. There is considerable controversy about how to best measure fibrosis. Liver biopsy and histology, long considered to be the gold standard, is invasive, and may be subject to sampling error.[47] Clinical methods (use of physical findings and routine laboratory tests such as platelets alone) are typically insensitive and not specific. A plethora of blood based test algorithms and serum markers of fibrosis (ie, TIMP1, MMP2, collagen I, III, IV, hyaluronic acid, and others) have been developed and studied extensively in patients with hepatitis C virus. Several have also been examined in HBV. The bulk of the data suggest that these tests have a high sensitivity and specificity for detection of far advanced fibrosis and cirrhosis, but are not highly sensitive or specific for less advanced stages of fibrosis.[48] Additionally, several imaging modalities, in particular vibration control transient elastography (also simply transient elastography) and magnetic resonance elastography are attractive to stage fibrosis because they are noninvasive. Like blood tests and serum marker panels, they are best for advanced fibrosis and cirrhosis, and less sensitive and specific for intermediate degrees of fibrosis.[48] It is clear that more research will be required in the area of monitoring of fibrosis regression.

Antifibrotic Therapy

Since the degree of liver fibrosis appears to be linked to the complications of chronic liver disease, including impaired synthetic function, liver failure, and perhaps hepatocellular cancer, is likely highly desirable to treat fibrosis as a primary endpoint. Fibrosis also appears to be tightly linked to portal hypertension, further justifying its primary treatment. Although attempts have been made previously to specifically treat the "fibrosis" component of liver disease, these approaches have generally been unsuccessful (see[1,4] for review). Thus, fibrosis represents a major unmet need in the field.

As highlighted, the most effective "antifibrotic" therapies are clearly those that treat or remove the underlying stimulus to fibrogenesis. With highly active and effective nucleos(t)ide analogs, this issue is important. Not only would it be expected for an antifibrotic agent to have beneficial effects in this population, but certain mechanistic approaches might be particularly attractive. For example, a compound that affects collagen cross-linking that might break down formed fibrous tissue, such as lysyl oxidase-like-2,[49] is attractive.

Reversion of Fibrosis and Outcomes with Viral Suppression

Abundant evidence in the HBV field indicates that treatment of patients with advanced fibrosis and cirrhosis—and with complications of HBV cirrhosis, including with esophageal varices, ascites, hepatic encephalopathy, and coagulopathy—with nucleos(t)ide analogs improves outcomes.[10,50–56] The evidence that this is related to fibrosis reversion is correlative, but is supported by data that indicate that treatment of patients with nucleos(t)ide analogs not only reduces fibrosis, but also has effects on portal hypertension. Notwithstanding, it is important to recognize that, even though fibrosis may be improved, the pathologic deposition of extracellular matrix and subsequent alteration in sinusoids and in blood flow may not necessarily be reversed. Because outcomes seem to be most closely tied to portal hypertension, this point is critical.

The natural history of HBV cirrhosis suggests that, after the development of complications, prognosis is poor, with a 5-year survival of approximately 25%. In contrast, although the long-term mortality in patients with complications of HBV cirrhosis after treatment with an oral HBV antiviral agent is not entirely clear, the 1-year survival for these patients is typically greater than 80% and may be greater than 90%.[50–56] Essentially, all of the currently used oral antiviral agents (lamivudine, adefovir, entecavir, telbivudine, or tenofovir) have been shown to lead to improved prognosis in patients with HBV and decompensated cirrhosis.

Although the studies examining HBV mediated decompensated cirrhosis have had different designs and have used different antivirals, the data suggest the following: (1) the oral antiviral agents all seem to be safe and effective, (2) clinical improvements in some patients have been such that some patients have been removed from liver transplant wait lists, (3) it has generally been recommended that, because of the infrequency of development of resistance, entecavir and tenofovir are the best choices for treatment of patients with HBV and decompensated cirrhosis, (4) all cirrhotic patients with decompensation should be treated, regardless of HBV DNA level as early as possible, and (5) oral agents (lamivudine, adefovir, entecavir, telbivudine, or tenofovir) are generally well-tolerated without significant side effects. Again, although these specific studies have focused on clinical endpoints and have generally not proven that there is a reversal of fibrosis/cirrhosis, the correlation between a change in fibrosis and outcome seems to be robust.

Further evidence of the benefit of HBV antiviral agents comes from large population studies. From 1985 to 2006, which coincided with the introduction of HBV antiviral agents, of 4793 patients with HBV cirrhosis wait listed for liver transplant, compared with 40,923 patients with hepatitis C virus cirrhosis, and 68,211 with neither type of viral disease, the decrease in incidence of waiting list registration was most pronounced for HBV cirrhosis.[57] Further, the increase in listing for hepatocellular carcinoma associated with HBV was least dramatic. These data suggested that the widespread use of oral antiviral therapy for HBV contributed to the decreased incidence of decompensated liver disease.

Despite the remarkable results in treating HBV cirrhosis patients with oral agents, there are some patients in whom the disease is too far advanced to expect a benefit. However, the clinical variables associated with a lack of response are currently unknown. Thus, it is this author's opinion that all patients with cirrhosis should be treated.

The Risk of Hepatocellular Carcinoma After Viral Suppression

Cirrhosis seems to be the most important risk factor for development of hepatocellular carcinoma. As such, reversal of fibrosis and cirrhosis would be expected to reduce the risk of development of hepatocellular carcinoma. In a large randomized trial of patients with HBV and advanced fibrosis (Ishak stage $\geq$4) who received lamivudine or placebo, 3.9% of patients receiving lamivudine and 7.4% of those receiving placebo developed hepatocellular carcinoma ($P = .047$), suggesting that viral suppression and reversal of fibrosis can prevent the development of hepatocellular carcinoma. Other studies, including metaanalyses, have suggested a similar decrease in the risk of development of hepatocellular carcinoma.[58–61] Although the risk of development of hepatocellular carcinoma seems to be low in certain patients with viral clearance (the strongest evidence seems to be in Asian patients), this affect does not seem to be uniform. For example, in a study of entecavir for treatment of HBV including 744 total patients and 164 patients with cirrhosis, over a median follow-up of 167 weeks, 14 patients developed hepatocellular carcinoma of whom 9 (64%) had cirrhosis at baseline. The 5-year cumulative incidence rate of hepatocellular carcinoma was 2.1% for noncirrhotic and 10.9% for cirrhotic patients (P<.001). Further, Caucasian patients seemed to maintain the highest hepatocellular carcinoma risk.[62]

SUMMARY

Great strides have been made in HBV-related fibrosis and cirrhosis. Currently, the evidence indicates that HBV viral suppression causes regression of advanced fibrosis and even cirrhosis in some patients, and therefore should be attempted in all patients with advanced fibrosis and cirrhosis. The preferred agents in patients with cirrhosis are entecavir and tenofovir, primarily because the risk of breakthrough is low. HBV viral suppression also leads to improved clinical outcomes even in patients with cirrhosis and complications (esophageal varices, ascites, hepatic encephalopathy, and coagulopathy). The risk of subsequent development of hepatocellular carcinoma is reduced after viral suppression, particularly in Asian patients, but less so in Caucasian patients. Thus, patients with HBV cirrhosis should continue to have routine screening for hepatocellular carcinoma, even after viral suppression.

REFERENCES

1. Rockey DC, Bell PD, Hill JA. Fibrosis–a common pathway to organ injury and failure. N Engl J Med 2015;372(12):1138–49.
2. Lozano R, Naghavi M, Foreman K, et al. Global and regional mortality from 235 causes of death for 20 age groups in 1990 and 2010: a systematic analysis for the Global Burden of Disease Study 2010. Lancet 2012;380(9859):2095–128.
3. Iredale JP, Benyon RC, Pickering J, et al. Mechanisms of spontaneous resolution of rat liver fibrosis. Hepatic stellate cell apoptosis and reduced hepatic expression of metalloproteinase inhibitors. J Clin Invest 1998;102(3):538–49.
4. Rockey DC. Translating an understanding of the pathogenesis of hepatic fibrosis to novel therapies. Clin Gastroenterol Hepatol 2013;11(3):224–31.e1-5.
5. Rockey DC. Antifibrotic therapy in chronic liver disease. Clin Gastroenterol Hepatol 2005;3(2):95–107.
6. Rockey DC, Chung JJ. Endothelin antagonism in experimental hepatic fibrosis. Implications for endothelin in the pathogenesis of wound healing. J Clin Invest 1996;98(6):1381–8.
7. Ellis EL, Mann DA. Clinical evidence for the regression of liver fibrosis. J Hepatol 2012;56(5):1171–80.
8. Crespo-Leiro MG, Robles O, Paniagua MJ, et al. Reversal of cardiac cirrhosis following orthotopic heart transplantation. Am J Transplant 2008;8(6):1336–9.
9. Czaja AJ, Carpenter HA. Decreased fibrosis during corticosteroid therapy of autoimmune hepatitis. J Hepatol 2004;40(4):646–52.
10. Liaw YF, Sung JJ, Chow WC, et al. Lamivudine for patients with chronic hepatitis B and advanced liver disease. N Engl J Med 2004;351(15):1521–31.
11. El-Husseini R, Kaplan MM. Reversal of portal hypertension in a patient with primary biliary cirrhosis: disappearance of esophageal varices and thrombocytopenia. Am J Gastroenterol 2004;99(9):1859–60.
12. Hammel P, Couvelard A, O'Toole D, et al. Regression of liver fibrosis after biliary drainage in patients with chronic pancreatitis and stenosis of the common bile duct. N Engl J Med 2001;344(6):418–23.
13. Wanless IR, Nakashima E, Sherman M. Regression of human cirrhosis. Morphologic features and the genesis of incomplete septal cirrhosis. Arch Pathol Lab Med 2000;124(11):1599–607.

14. Dufour JF, DeLellis R, Kaplan MM. Reversibility of hepatic fibrosis in autoimmune hepatitis. Ann Intern Med 1997;127(11):981–5.
15. Kweon YO, Goodman ZD, Dienstag JL, et al. Decreasing fibrogenesis: an immunohistochemical study of paired liver biopsies following lamivudine therapy for chronic hepatitis B. J Hepatol 2001;35(6):749–55.
16. Chang TT, Liaw YF, Wu SS, et al. Long-term entecavir therapy results in the reversal of fibrosis/cirrhosis and continued histological improvement in patients with chronic hepatitis B. Hepatology 2010;52(3):886–93.
17. Marcellin P, Gane E, Buti M, et al. Regression of cirrhosis during treatment with tenofovir disoproxil fumarate for chronic hepatitis B: a 5-year open-label follow-up study. Lancet 2013;381(9865):468–75.
18. Liaw YF. Reversal of cirrhosis: an achievable goal of hepatitis B antiviral therapy. J Hepatol 2013;59(4):880–1.
19. Shiratori Y, Imazeki F, Moriyama M, et al. Histologic improvement of fibrosis in patients with hepatitis C who have sustained response to interferon therapy. Ann Intern Med 2000;132(7):517–24.
20. Poynard T, McHutchison J, Manns M, et al. Impact of pegylated interferon alfa-2b and ribavirin on liver fibrosis in patients with chronic hepatitis C. Gastroenterology 2002;122(5):1303–13.
21. Mallet V, Gilgenkrantz H, Serpaggi J, et al. Brief communication: the relationship of regression of cirrhosis to outcome in chronic hepatitis C. Ann Intern Med 2008; 149(6):399–403.
22. Farci P, Roskams T, Chessa L, et al. Long-term benefit of interferon alpha therapy of chronic hepatitis D: regression of advanced hepatic fibrosis. Gastroenterology 2004;126(7):1740–9.
23. Powell LW, Kerr JF. Reversal of "cirrhosis" in idiopathic haemochromatosis following long-term intensive venesection therapy. Australas Ann Med 1970; 19(1):54–7.
24. Blumberg RS, Chopra S, Ibrahim R, et al. Primary hepatocellular carcinoma in idiopathic hemochromatosis after reversal of cirrhosis. Gastroenterology 1988; 95(5):1399–402.
25. Sorensen TI, Orholm M, Bentsen KD, et al. Prospective evaluation of alcohol abuse and alcoholic liver injury in men as predictors of development of cirrhosis. Lancet 1984;2(8397):241–4.
26. Berhe N, Myrvang B, Gundersen SG. Reversibility of schistosomal periportal thickening/fibrosis after praziquantel therapy: a twenty-six month follow-up study in Ethiopia. Am J Trop Med Hyg 2008;78(2):228–34.
27. Sohara N, Znoyko I, Levy MT, et al. Reversal of activation of human myofibroblast-like cells by culture on a basement membrane-like substrate. J Hepatol 2002; 37(2):214–21.
28. Deleve LD, Wang X, Guo Y. Sinusoidal endothelial cells prevent rat stellate cell activation and promote reversion to quiescence. Hepatology 2008;48(3):920–30.
29. Troeger JS, Mederacke I, Gwak GY, et al. Deactivation of hepatic stellate cells during liver fibrosis resolution in mice. Gastroenterology 2012;143(4): 1073–83.e22.
30. Iredale JP. Stellate cell behavior during resolution of liver injury. Semin Liver Dis 2001;21(3):427–36.
31. Preaux AM, D'Ortho MP, Bralet MP, et al. Apoptosis of human hepatic myofibroblasts promotes activation of matrix metalloproteinase-2. Hepatology 2002;36(3): 615–22.

32. Li L, Tao J, Davaille J, et al. 15-deoxy-Delta 12,14-prostaglandin J2 induces apoptosis of human hepatic myofibroblasts. A pathway involving oxidative stress independently of peroxisome-proliferator-activated receptors. J Biol Chem 2001; 276(41):38152–8.

33. Thoen LF, Guimaraes EL, Grunsven LA. Autophagy: a new player in hepatic stellate cell activation. Autophagy 2012;8(1):126–8.

34. Thoen LF, Guimaraes EL, Dolle L, et al. A role for autophagy during hepatic stellate cell activation. J Hepatol 2011;55(6):1353–60.

35. Hernndez-Gea V, Friedman SL. Autophagy fuels tissue fibrogenesis. Autophagy 2012;8(5):849–50.

36. Hernandez-Gea V, Ghiassi-Nejad Z, Rozenfeld R, et al. Autophagy releases lipid that promotes fibrogenesis by activated hepatic stellate cells in mice and in human tissues. Gastroenterology 2012;142(4):938–46.

37. Schnabl B, Purbeck CA, Choi YH, et al. Replicative senescence of activated human hepatic stellate cells is accompanied by a pronounced inflammatory but less fibrogenic phenotype. Hepatology 2003;37(3):653–64.

38. Krizhanovsky V, Yon M, Dickins RA, et al. Senescence of activated stellate cells limits liver fibrosis. Cell 2008;134(4):657–67.

39. Kong X, Feng D, Wang H, et al. Interleukin-22 induces hepatic stellate cell senescence and restricts liver fibrosis in mice. Hepatology 2012;56(3):1150–9.

40. Marcellin P, Asselah T. Long-term therapy for chronic hepatitis B: hepatitis B virus DNA suppression leading to cirrhosis reversal. J Gastroenterol Hepatol 2013; 28(6):912–23.

41. Dienstag JL, Goldin RD, Heathcote EJ, et al. Histological outcome during long-term lamivudine therapy. Gastroenterology 2003;124(1):105–17.

42. Rizzetto M, Tassopoulos NC, Goldin RD, et al. Extended lamivudine treatment in patients with HBeAg-negative chronic hepatitis B. J Hepatol 2005;42(2):173–9.

43. Hadziyannis SJ, Tassopoulos NC, Heathcote EJ, et al. Long-term therapy with adefovir dipivoxil for HBeAg-negative chronic hepatitis B for up to 5 years. Gastroenterology 2006;131(6):1743–51.

44. Marcellin P, Chang TT, Lim SG, et al. Long-term efficacy and safety of adefovir dipivoxil for the treatment of hepatitis B e antigen-positive chronic hepatitis B. Hepatology 2008;48(3):750–8.

45. Schiff E, Simsek H, Lee WM, et al. Efficacy and safety of entecavir in patients with chronic hepatitis B and advanced hepatic fibrosis or cirrhosis. Am J Gastroenterol 2008;103(11):2776–83.

46. Yokosuka O, Takaguchi K, Fujioka S, et al. Long-term use of entecavir in nucleoside-naive Japanese patients with chronic hepatitis B infection. J Hepatol 2010;52(6):791–9.

47. Rockey DC, Caldwell SH, Goodman ZD, et al. Liver biopsy. Hepatology 2009; 49(3):1017–44.

48. Rockey DC, Bissell DM. Noninvasive measures of liver fibrosis. Hepatology 2006; 43(2 Suppl 1):S113–20.

49. Barry-Hamilton V, Spangler R, Marshall D, et al. Allosteric inhibition of lysyl oxidase-like-2 impedes the development of a pathologic microenvironment. Nat Med 2010;16(9):1009–17.

50. Fontana RJ, Hann HW, Perrillo RP, et al. Determinants of early mortality in patients with decompensated chronic hepatitis B treated with antiviral therapy. Gastroenterology 2002;123(3):719–27.

51. Schiff ER, Lai CL, Hadziyannis S, et al. Adefovir dipivoxil therapy for lamivudine-resistant hepatitis B in pre- and post-liver transplantation patients. Hepatology 2003;38(6):1419–27.
52. Shim JH, Lee HC, Kim KM, et al. Efficacy of entecavir in treatment-naive patients with hepatitis B virus-related decompensated cirrhosis. J Hepatol 2010;52(2): 176–82.
53. Liaw YF, Raptopoulou-Gigi M, Cheinquer H, et al. Efficacy and safety of entecavir versus adefovir in chronic hepatitis B patients with hepatic decompensation: a randomized, open-label study. Hepatology 2011;54(1):91–100.
54. Liaw YF, Sheen IS, Lee CM, et al. Tenofovir disoproxil fumarate (TDF), emtricitabine/TDF, and entecavir in patients with decompensated chronic hepatitis B liver disease. Hepatology 2011;53(1):62–72.
55. Chan HL, Chen YC, Gane EJ, et al. Randomized clinical trial: efficacy and safety of telbivudine and lamivudine in treatment-naive patients with HBV-related decompensated cirrhosis. J Viral Hepat 2012;19(10):732–43.
56. Zoutendijk R, Reijnders JG, Zoulim F, et al. Virological response to entecavir is associated with a better clinical outcome in chronic hepatitis B patients with cirrhosis. Gut 2013;62(5):760–5.
57. Kim WR, Terrault NA, Pedersen RA, et al. Trends in waiting list registration for liver transplantation for viral hepatitis in the United States. Gastroenterology 2009; 137(5):1680–6.
58. Matsumoto A, Tanaka E, Rokuhara A, et al. Efficacy of lamivudine for preventing hepatocellular carcinoma in chronic hepatitis B: a multicenter retrospective study of 2795 patients. Hepatol Res 2005;32(3):173–84.
59. Miyake Y, Kobashi H, Yamamoto K. Meta-analysis: the effect of interferon on development of hepatocellular carcinoma in patients with chronic hepatitis B virus infection. J Gastroenterol 2009;44(5):470–5.
60. Papatheodoridis GV, Lampertico P, Manolakopoulos S, et al. Incidence of hepatocellular carcinoma in chronic hepatitis B patients receiving nucleos(t)ide therapy: a systematic review. J Hepatol 2010;53(2):348–56.
61. Papatheodoridis GV, Manolakopoulos S, Touloumi G, et al. Virological suppression does not prevent the development of hepatocellular carcinoma in HBeAg-negative chronic hepatitis B patients with cirrhosis receiving oral antiviral(s) starting with lamivudine monotherapy: results of the nationwide HEPNET. Greece cohort study. Gut 2011;60(8):1109–16.
62. Arends P, Sonneveld MJ, Zoutendijk R, et al. Entecavir treatment does not eliminate the risk of hepatocellular carcinoma in chronic hepatitis B: limited role for risk scores in Caucasians. Gut 2015;64(8):1289–95.

Hepatitis B Virus Infection and Liver Decompensation

Brendon K. Luvisa, BA[a], Tarek I. Hassanein, MD[a,b],*

KEYWORDS

- Hepatitis B virus • Hepatocellular carcinoma • Highly active antivirals
- Liver decompensation • Liver support system

KEY POINTS

- The goal in patients with immune active hepatitis B virus (HBV) infection is to significantly suppress viral replication and prevent progression of fibrosis to cirrhosis and liver decompensation and decrease the incidence of hepatocellular carcinoma (HCC).
- This is achievable by the highly active antivirals, entecavir and tenofovir, which are considered the first line of therapy in most patients with immune active hepatitis C virus and after liver transplantation to prevent HBV recurrence.
- The existing data have some limitations due to the heterogenetic patient population involved in studies.
- Recent attempts to use liver support systems to help bridge the patients to recovery from the acute episode of liver failure or to liver transplantation showed some encouraging results but need more confirmation in well-designed multicenter studies.

INTRODUCTION

Hepatitis B virus (HBV) is a double-stranded DNA virus with high level of infectivity. It is prevalent among all populations of the world. The global prevalence of chronic hepatitis B is approximately 5%. It is estimated to have infected more than 2 billion people around the world. The impact of the viral infection is still seen in many countries, in the form of chronic hepatitis, liver cirrhosis, and liver cancer. Since the introduction of HBV vaccine in 1982, and with the strict implementation of vaccination, many countries had been able to prevent new infections in the newborn and children. Despite all efforts, there are more than 240 million chronic carriers of the virus, most of whom are in the Asian Pacific region.[1]

Chronically infected patients could develop progressive chronic hepatitis, progressive fibrosis to cirrhosis with subsequent liver decompensation, resulting in death unless treated timely or undergo liver transplantation. In addition, HBV chronic infection

The authors have nothing to disclose.
[a] Southern California Research Center, Coronado, CA 92118, USA; [b] University of California, San Diego School of Medicine, San Diego, CA, USA
* Corresponding author. Southern California Research Center, Coronado, CA 92118.
E-mail address: thassanein@livercenters.com

Clin Liver Dis 20 (2016) 681–692
http://dx.doi.org/10.1016/j.cld.2016.07.002
1089-3261/16/© 2016 Elsevier Inc. All rights reserved.

liver.theclinics.com

increases the chances of developing liver cancer even in patients without cirrhosis. It is estimated to have to be 0.5 to 1.2 million annual deaths per year from HBV infection.[1]

HBV is transmitted parenterally via percutaneous or per-mucosal exposure to infected blood or body fluids. Once infection occurs in a patient who is not vaccinated, the virus may induce acute hepatitis B, which could be clinically evident or subclinically unnoticed. Although most adult patients will recover from an acute infection by developing acquired immunity, producing HBsAb (Hepatitis B Surface Antibody), fewer than 10% of patients will develop chronic HBV infection in adults.[2] During the acute phase, a very small number (<1%) of patients will develop acute fulminant hepatitis B and liver failure.[3] In contrast, perinatal or early childhood infection always results in chronic infection, unless newborns receive their vaccine and/or HBV immunoglobulin within the early hours of their lives.[4]

Hepatitis B has 8 to 10 different genotypes with different prevalence in the world; genotype A is in the United States and western Europe, genotypes B and C are in Asia, genotype D is most prevalent in the Mediterranean region, E in Africa, and F and H in South America and Mexico.[5-8] Genotypes have an impact on the natural history of the disease and on response to therapy. Precore mutations are reported more often in genotype D than in C and B, respectively, and HBeAg-negative CHB (Hepatitis B E Antigen-negative Chronic Hepatitis B) is more common in the Middle East region than in the United States and western Europe.[9]

NATURAL HISTORY

HBV infection in infants at birth results in 90% rate of developing chronic infection, which decreases to 20% to 30% if infection occurs in children aged 1 to 5 years, and the chronicity rate drops to 6% in children 5 to 15 years of age, and is less than 5% in adult patients. In the acute phase, particularly in adults, the liver rarely decompensates in the form of fulminant hepatic failure where an overwhelming immune response occurs against the infected hepatocytes, causing massive liver cell death and presenting clinically in acute liver failure, and is associated with greater than 70% mortality. However, the great majority of acute infections may pass clinically unnoticed in infected individuals.[4]

Patients who develop chronic infection present in different disease phases. These distinct phases result from the interaction of the virus with the host-immune response and other viral coinfections.[2,4] Infection in infancy and early childhood present in 1 of 3 phases: immune-tolerant phase, inactive carrier state, or spontaneous seroconversion. Later in life many of the actively infected patients develop HBeAg-positive CHB, and progress to HBeAg-negative CHB. In contrast, adult-acquired chronic HBV infection goes through the HBeAg-positive phase that might seroconvert over time to HBeAg-negative phase and develop HBe-Ab; however, they do not develop the initial immune-tolerant phase seen in infants and children.[10] When patients go through the phase of spontaneous seroconversion of HBeAg or HBsAg they occasionally present with an exacerbation of hepatitis, which on rare occasion could be severe enough to cause acute liver failure or liver decompensation.[11-17]

Fourteen percent to 30% of patients with chronic HBV develop cirrhosis and complications of end-stage liver disease. Active viral replication, alcohol consumption, or coinfection with hepatitis C virus (HCV) or human immunodeficiency virus (HIV) increases the risk of hepatic decompensation.[18] In a European longitudinal study of 366 patients followed for a mean period of 72 months, death occurred in 23% of patients either from liver failure or hepatocellular carcinoma (HCC).[19] Survival correlated with age, albumin levels, platelet count, bilirubin levels, presence of splenomegaly, and HBeAg positivity.[20] The 5-year probability of hepatic decompensation in patients with HBeAg-positive HBV cirrhosis is 15% to 20% and is usually more seen in patients with active viral replication.[21,22]

Decompensation in the setting of cirrhosis decreases 5-year survival rate to 30% to 50%.[1–22] HCV coinfection or superinfection has been reported to increase the risk of severe hepatitis and fulminant hepatic failure.[23–25] A similar presentation is seen with HDV (Hepatitis D Virus) superinfection and occasionally with HEV (Hepatitis E Virus) superinfection in patients with cirrhosis.[26,27]

HEPATIC DECOMPENSATION

Liver decompensation presents in the form of progressive development of ascites, jaundice, or encephalopathy or after a variceal bleed.[28,29] It occurs as part of the natural progression of chronic HBV infection in the setting of cirrhosis, or as a result of HBV reactivation and acute hepatitis flare.[22] It is reported that HBV flare in the setting of cirrhosis results in an estimated 14% decompensation.[30] Decompensation is always seen in the presence of HBV-DNA positivity. It is more commonly seen in HBeAg-positive patients than HBeAg-negative patients.[21,31]

In an Asian study of 96 patients over a period of 3 years, decompensation occurred in 29% of the patients and presented as ascites in 70%, variceal bleeding in 34%, jaundice in 26%, and hepatic encephalopathy in 5.2% of the patients; 29% had more than one feature of decompensation. The causes of death were hepatic failure in 52.9%, HCC in 29.4%, variceal bleeding in 5.9%, and SBP (Spontaneous Bacterial Peritonitis) in 4.4%.[32] Similar findings were reported in another study of 102 patients, where the presenting clinical feature of decompensation was ascites in 63% and variceal bleeding in 37% of the patients. The mean 5-year survival rate was 19%. The cause of death was hepatorenal syndrome in 32%, variceal bleeding in 23%, HCC in 28%, liver failure in 9%, and hepatic encephalopathy in 9%.[33]

ACUTE ON CHRONIC LIVER FAILURE

Acute on chronic liver failure (AoCLF) is considered in patients with chronic HBV who sustain an acute liver insult resulting in jaundice, coagulopathy, ascites, and/or encephalopathy. AoCLF is associated with high mortality rate. Reactivation of HBV presenting with significant elevation of transaminases, jaundice, ascites, and liver cell failure is a form of AoCLF. AoCLF is also seen with viral superinfection (HDV, HCV, HEV), acute variceal bleeding, bacteria peritonitis, sepsis, and acute alcoholic hepatitis. In AoCLF and Model for End-Stage Liver Disease (MELD) score greater than 20, even in the presence of viral suppression, the 3-month mortality is still high (50%).[34–36]

In a recent meta-analysis of 4 studies addressing patients with chronic HBV infection experiencing AoCLF, antiviral therapy using lamivudine, entecavir, telbivudine, or tenofovir reduced all-cause mortality (Relative Risk (RR) = 0.7, 95% confidence interval 0.6–0.8, I^2 = 5.4%).[35,37–40]

NATURAL HISTORY AFTER HEPATIC DECOMPENSATION

Hepatic decompensation signifies low survival rates. The 5-year survival rate is 14% to 35% compared with 85% reported for compensated patients.[31] Mortality results from complications of decompensation and liver cell failure such as development of SIRS (Systemic Inflammatory Response Syndrome) or sepsis, SBP, HRS (Hepatorenal Syndrome), or from advanced liver cancer. Two major scores have been routinely used to estimate mortality in patients with liver decompensation. The Child-Pugh-Turcotte

(CPT) score, which predicts 1-year survival, and the MELD score, which predicts short-term mortality (**Tables 1** and **2**).[41,42] The recent ACLF-CLIF score (Acute-on-Chronic Liver Failure- Chronic Liver Failure) was introduced to predict short-term mortality in patients with AoCLF.[43]

MANAGEMENT OF HEPATIC DECOMPENSATION IN THE SETTING OF HEPATITIS B VIRUS INFECTION

Standard care in patients with HBV-associated liver decompensation starts with detailed investigation of the stage of HBV, the presence of any 2 viral coinfections, and addressing the signs of decompensation, such as ascites, esophageal varices, renal dysfunction, hepatic encephalopathy, coagulopathy, presence of sepsis or SIRS, and HCC. Immediate management is directed toward controlling factors inducing liver decompensation, starting with viral suppression and management of any infection. Early liver transplant evaluation is crucial, particularly in patients who decompensated as a result of other viral superinfections or other underlying comorbidities.[44,45]

ANTIVIRAL DRUG THERAPY

Chronic HBV infection is a noncurable infection, because the virus continues to be detected in the liver cells even after clearance of HBsAg and the development of anti-HBs.[46] Residual cccDNA (covalently closed circular DNA) of the virus continues to persist in the liver cells even with long-term suppressive therapy. HBV-DNA sequence integrates into the hepatocyte genomes and is not eliminated before hepatocyte death.[47] Attempts to eradicate HBV and its cccDNA is currently under investigation (see Sebastien Boucle and colleagues' article, "Towards Elimination of Hepatitis B Virus Using Novel Drugs, Approaches, and Combined Modalities," elsewhere in this issue).

However, suppression of HBV-DNA and HBsAg seroconversion continue to be the ultimate goals of currently availably therapies (Functional Cure). Achieving viral suppression is associated in most patients with normalization of transaminases, improvement in hepatocyte function, improvement in albumin levels and international

Table 1
The Child-Pugh-Turcotte Score and its score interpretation

Child-Pugh-Turcotte Score (CPT)[41]			
Measure	1 Point	2 Points	3 Points
Total bilirubin, μmol/L (mg/dL)	<34 (<2)	34–50[2,3]	>50 (>3)
Serum albumin, g/dL	>3.5	2.8–3.5	<2.8
Prothrombin time, prolongation(s)	<4.0	4.0–6.0	> 6.0
Ascites	None	Mild	Moderate to severe
Hepatic encephalopathy	None	Grade I–II (or suppressed with medication)	Grade III–IV (or refractory)

CPT Score Interpretation			
Points	Class	One-Year Survival, %	Two-Year Survival, %
5–6	A	100	85
7–9	B	81	57
10–15	C	45	35

Table 2
MELD score and interpretation

MELD Score	3-mo Mortality Risk, %
22	10
29	30
33	50
38	80

Model for End-Stage Liver Disease (MELD) formula: MELD = 3.78 × ln(serum bilirubin [mg/dL]) + 11.2 × ln(INR) + 9.57 × ln(serum creatinine [mg/dL]) + 6.43.
Data from Kamat PS, Wiesner RH, Malinchoc M, et al. A model to predict survival in patients with end-stage liver disease. Hepatology 2001;33:464–70.

normalized ratio (INR), and reversal of liver decompensation; and some patients had reversal of fibrosis even at the stage of early cirrhosis.[48]

Studies of compensated patients with HBV-related cirrhosis who are untreated have a 5-year survival rate of 80% to 85% versus 14% to 25% for those with decompensated cirrhosis.[18,19,22,32] Kim and colleagues in a retrospective study in a Korean cohort of 240 patients, reported 5-year probability of survival of 56% in the untreated historical cohort. If patients were classified by CPT, the 5-year survival was 74.3% in CPT-A 33.5% in CPT-B, and 10.2% for CPT-C. With antiviral therapy, the overall 5-year survival was 80.6%, and was 90.9%, 62.8%, and 62.2% for CPT-A, CPT-B, and CPT-C, respectively. The study showed 15.4% probability of hepatic decompensation in 5 years after starting antiviral treatment and 13.8% probability of developing HCC.[49]

THERAPY OF PATIENTS WITH HEPATITIS B VIRUS WITH LIVER DECOMPENSATION

Most studies showed that suppression of HBV viral replication in patients with HBV-related cirrhosis prevents the deterioration of liver cell function and reduces the incidence of liver decompensation and HCC and improves the overall survival of patients. Antiviral therapy should be started immediately in any viremic patients with HBV-decompensated cirrhosis regardless of serum HBV-DNA levels (**Table 3**).

Table 3
First-line antivirals in decompensated HBV cirrhosis

Authors, Reference, y	Antiviral Drug	Duration of Therapy, mo	CPT Score at Entry	Decrease CPT ≥2 Points, %	HBV-DNA Undetectable, %	LT, %	Overall Survival, %
Shim et al,[56] 2010	ETV	12	≥7	49	93	4	90
Liaw et al,[57] 2011	ETV	24	≥7	35	57	11	82
Liaw et al,[58] 2011	ETV	12	7–12	42	73	0	91
Liaw et al,[58] 2011	TDV	12	7–12	26	71	4	96
Liaw et al,[58] 2011	TRU	12	7–12	48	88	9	96

Abbreviations: CPT, Child-Pugh-Turcotte; ETV, entecavir; HBV, hepatitis B virus; LT, liver transplantation; TDV, tenofovir; TRU, truvada (emtricitabine and tenofovir disoproxil fumarate).

Lamivudine was the first HBV antiviral approved and used in patients with HBV-related cirrhosis and decompensation. Lamivudine was very effective in the short term; however, due to the progressive increase in rates of viral resistance (20% at year 1 and up to 80% at year 5), it fell out of favor as first line of therapy.[50,51] Similar challenges with resistance were encountered with adefovir (29% resistance at year 5) and telbivudine (resistance >20% at year 2).[52,53] Currently, entecavir and tenofovir are considered the first line of therapy due to their safety, efficacy, and minimal to no risk of resistance in naïve patients.[45,54,55] However, in lamivudine-resistant patients, entecavir is not recommended due to a 35% to 50% chance of developing HBV resistance after 5 years of therapy and in decompensated patients it rarely induces lactic acidosis. In these patients, tenofovir is considered the drug of choice. Long-term use of tenofovir is known to cause renal impairment, including Fanconi anemia, hypophosphatemia, and osteopenia in patients with HIV infection and it is recommended to monitor patients on long-term tenofovir therapy for the same complications. A recent meta-analysis comparing the 2 drugs did not show significant difference in renal function and serum phosphate during therapy.[55]

Shim and colleagues reported on 70 decompensated patients treated with entecavir. After 12 months of therapy, 89% of decompensated patients had undetectable HBV-DNA and 22% had HBe-Ag seroconversion; however, 6 patients died, 3 patients had liver transplantation, and 5 patients developed HCC.[56] Liaw and colleagues reported on 100 patients with liver decompensation who were treated with entecavir; 57% had undetectable HBV by their assay by week 48. Eleven patients underwent liver transplantation and their reported overall survival was 82%[57] (see **Table 3**). Jang and colleagues reported on 707 patients with HBV-related decompensation who were followed for 7 years. They reported 5-year transplant-free survival of 59.7%. In their patients with severe hepatic dysfunction, 13.4% died within the first 6 months of therapy. They showed effectiveness of long-term viral suppression and its benefit in delaying or negating the need for liver transplantation in 60% of their transplant-eligible cohort. They were able to delist 33.9% of the liver transplant–listed patients within 1 year. Their study underscored the long-term benefit of viral suppression on the natural history of patients with decompensated cirrhosis and improvement in transplant-free survival.[59] Cholongitas and colleagues in a retrospective study, reported on 52 patients with HBV-related cirrhosis and decompensation receiving either tenofovir (n = 31) or entecavir (n = 21) and were followed for 22.5 months. All patients had undetectable serum HBV-DNA at 12 months and at end of follow-up. All remained HBeAg-negative and none had HBsAg clearance. Nine (17%) patients either died (n = 3) or received transplantation (n = 6). Death resulted from sepsis in 2 patients and HCC in 1 patient. In a multivariable Cox regression analysis of the group of patients without HCC, changes and CPT and MELD score from baseline to 6 months were significant ($P = .035$, $P = .031$, respectively) and independently associated with outcome.[60]

In the past decade, the use of antivirals in HBV-related liver decompensation resulted in improvement in hepatic function and in some patients' withdrawal from the liver transplant waiting list. Shim and colleagues reported a decrease in MELD score from 11.1 at baseline to 8.8 at 12 months on treatment in 49% of the patients receiving entecavir. The mean reduction in MELD was 2.3 points. The CPT score improved by 2 or more during the same period.[56] Liaw and colleagues reported on patients receiving entecavir or tenofovir or tenofovir/embtricitabine (FTC) an improvement in CPT score by 2 points in 26% to 48% of the patients, and their MELD score decreased by a median of 2 points at 12 months compared with baseline.[58] Peng and colleagues showed a mean of 2 points' improvement in MELD score in patients who responded to antiviral therapy.[61] Cholongitas and colleagues, in 52 patients treated by entecavir or tenofovir, showed similar responses to the previous studies with reduction in MELD score of 1.5 points from baseline and a decrease in the CPT score of 2 or more points in 21% of patients by 12 months of therapy.[60]

Most studies have shown high mortality in the first 6 months of therapy in patients with severe liver decompensation, and before complete viral suppression occurs.[59] Patients who continue to exhibit hepatic decompensation CPT class C or MELD score greater than or equal to 15, despite viral suppression, have a poor short-term prognosis and should pursue liver transplantation.

In a trial by Duan and colleagues using the ELAD system (a biological liver support system), 49 patients with chronic hepatitis B and acute liver decompensation from acute viral reactivation (AoCLF) were randomized into a controlled open-label trial at 2 hospitals in China to either receive the ELAD system treatment for 1 to 3 days in addition to standard of care versus standard of care alone. There was a significant difference in 28-day and 56-day survival using the log-rank test ($P = .015$ and .026, respectively), and the study reported no unexpected safety issues. Based on the preliminary results, it was concluded that the ELAD system should be further evaluated in more severely diseased populations with AoCLF as a salvage therapy or as a bridge to transplantation, and the treatment protocols should be extended more than 3 days.[62]

LIVER TRANSPLANTATION FOR PATIENTS INFECTED WITH HEPATITIS B

Patients with HBV-related liver decompensation should be referred for liver transplantation and maintained on a first-line antiviral to achieve full suppression of viral replication. Close monitoring and management of signs of decompensation is enforced. With full suppression of viral replications, the liver function recovers in 3 to 6 months and MELD score will improve in patients responding to therapy. The goal of therapy is to suppress the virus under 100,000 copies/mL before the transplant surgery to minimize recurrent rate after transplantation.[63] Decompensated patients who receive liver transplantation have a 5-year patient and graft survival rate of 75% and 71%, respectively, compared with patients with HBV-related HCC who received a liver transplant, whose 5-year patient and graft survival rates are lower at 68% and 65%, respectively.[64]

Recurrence after liver transplantation occurs in patients who had pretransplant HBV-DNA levels and those with viral mutations and patients with HCC.[65] Prevention of HBV recurrence after transplantation involves the use of hepatitis B immunoglobulin in combination with antivirals, depending on the viral status of the patient at the time of transplantation.[66–69]

In conclusion, the goal in patients with immune active HBV infection is to significantly suppress viral replication and prevent progression of fibrosis to cirrhosis and liver decompensation and decrease the incidence of HCC. This is achievable by the highly active antivirals, entecavir and tenofovir, which are considered the first line of therapy in most patients with immune active HCV and after liver transplantation to prevent HBV recurrence (**Fig. 1**).

However, the existing data have some limitations due to the heterogenetic patient population involved in studies. Most of the studies were short term with no long-term data, and some were retrospective. Patients presenting with AoCLF in the setting of viral replication have a high mortality rate and require liver transplantation. Recent attempts to use liver support systems to help bridge the patients to recovery from the acute episode of liver failure or to liver transplantation showed some encouraging results but need more confirmation in well-designed multicenter studies.

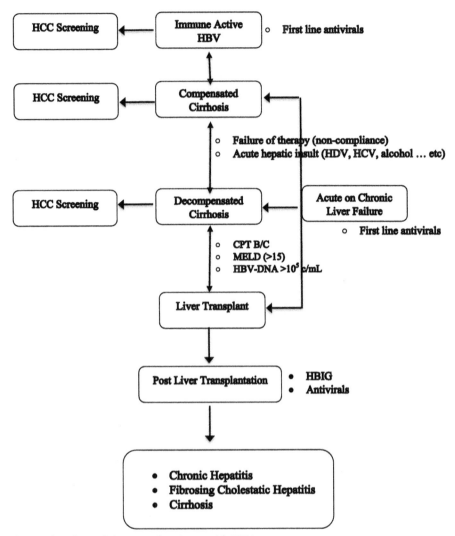

Fig. 1. Flowchart of therapy of patients with HBV.

Patients with advanced liver decompensation who in the presence of complete viral suppression still maintain a high MELD score (>15) have a poor prognosis without liver transplantation. Although entecavir and tenofovir have shown excellent safety and efficacy, their reported adverse events of lactic acidosis and renal injury should be monitored closely.

In summary, patients with decompensated cirrhosis should be referred for liver transplantation and treated with first-line antivirals as early as possible, with the goal of achieving complete viral suppression in the shortest time possible.

REFERENCES

1. Lavanchy D. Hepatitis B virus epidemiology, disease burden, treatment, and current and emerging prevention and control measures. J Viral Hepatol 2004;11:97–107.

2. Rehermann B, Ferrari C, Pasquinelli C, et al. The hepatitis B virus persists for decades after patients' recovery from acute viral hepatitis despite active maintenance of a cytotoxic T lymphocyte response. Nat Med 1996;2:1106–8.

3. Chu CM, Liaw YF. Increased incidence of fulminant hepatic failure in previously unrecognized HBsAg carriers with acute hepatitis independent of etiology. Infection 2005;33:136–9.

4. McMahon BJ, Alward WI, Hall DB, et al. Acute hepatitis B virus infection: relation of age to the clinical expression of disease and subsequent development of the carrier state. J Infect Dis 1985;151:599–603.

5. Kao JH. Role of viral factors in the natural course and therapy of chronic hepatitis B. Hepaol Int 2007;1:415–30.

6. Fung SK, Los AS. Hepatitis B virus genotypes: do they play a role in the outcome of HBV infection? Hepatology 2004;40(4):790–2.

7. Norder H, Courouce AM, Coursaget P, et al. Genetic diversity of hepatitis B virus strains derived worldwide: genotypes, subgenotypes, and HBsAg subtypes. Intervirology 2004;47(6):289–309.

8. Chu CJ, Keeffe EB, Han SH, et al. Hepatitis B virus genotypes in the Unites States: results of a nationwide study. Gastroenterology 2003;125(2):444–51.

9. Manesis EK. HBeAg-negative chronic hepatitis B: from obscurity to prominence. J Hepatol 2006;45:343–6.

10. Lai CL, Ratziu V, Yuen MF, et al. Viral hepatitis B. Lancet 2003;362:2089–94.

11. McMahon BJ. Epidemiology and natural history of hepatitis B. Semin Liver Dis 2005;25(Suppl 1):3–8.

12. Hoofnagle JH, Dusheiko GM, Seeff LB, et al. Seroconversion from hepatitis B e antigen to antibody in chronic type B hepatitis. Ann Intern Med 1981;94(6):744–8.

13. Fattovich G, Rugge M, Brollo L, et al. Clinical, virologic and histologic outcome following seroconversion from HBeAg to anti-HBe in chronic hepatitis type B. Hepatology 1986;6(2):167–72.

14. Lok AS, Lai CL, Wu PC, et al. Spontaneous hepatitis B e antigen to antibody seroconversion and reversion in Chinese patients with chronic hepatitis B virus infection. Gastroenterology 1987;92(6):1839–43.

15. Bortolotti F, Guido M, Bartolacci S, et al. Chronic hepatitis B in children after e antigen seroclearance: final report of a 29-year longitudinal study. Hepatology 2006;42(3):556–62.

16. McMahaon BJ, Holck P, Bulkow L, et al. Serologic and clinical outcomes of 1536 Alaska Natives chronically infected with hepatitis B virus. Ann Intern Med 2001;135(9):759–68.

17. Hsu YS, Chien RN, Yeh CT, et al. Long-term outcomes after spontaneous HBeAg seroconversion in patients with chronic hepatitis B. Hepatology 2002;35(6):1522–7.

18. Fattovich G, Bortolotti F, Donato F. Natural history of chronic hepatitis B: special emphasis on disease progression and prognostic factors. J Hepatol 2008;28(2):335–52.

19. Realdi G, Fattovich G, Hadziyannis S, et al. Survival and prognostic factors in 366 patients with compensated cirrhosis type B: a multicenter study. The Investigators of the European Concerted Action on Viral Hepatitis (EUROHEP). J Hepatol 1994;21(4):656–66.

20. Fontana RJ, Hann HW, Perillo RP, et al. Determinants of early mortality in patients with decompensated chronic hepatitis B treated with antiviral therapy. Gastroenterology 2002;123:719–27.

21. Chen YC, Chu CM, Yeh CT, et al. Natural course following the onset of cirrhosis in patients with chronic hepatitis B: a long-term follow-up study. Hepatol Int 2007;1: 267–73.

22. Chu CM, Liaw YF. Hepatitis B virus-related cirrhosis: natural history and treatment. Semin Liv Dis 2006;26:142–52.

23. Chu CM, Yeh CT, Liaw YF. Fulminant hepatitis failure in acute hepatitis C: increased risk in chronic carriers of hepatitis B virus. Gut 1999;45(4):613–7.

24. Liaw YF, Chen YC, Sheen IS, et al. Impact of acute hepatitis C virus superinfection in patients with chronic hepatitis B virus infection. Gastroenterology 2004;126(4): 1024–9.

25. Mimms LT, Mosley JW, Hollinger FB, et al. Effect of concurrent acute infection with hepatitis C virus on acute hepatitis B virus infection. MGJ 1993;307(6912): 1095–7.

26. Fattovich G, Boscaro S, Noventa F, et al. Influence of hepatitis delta virus infection on progression to cirrhosis in chronic hepatitis type B. J Infec Dis 1987;155(5): 931–5.

27. Fattovich G, Giustina G, Chistensen E, et al. Influence of hepatitis delta virus infection on morbidity and mortality in compensated cirrhosis type B. The European Concerted Action on Viral Hepatitis (Eurohep). Gut 2000;46(3):420–6.

28. Fattovich G, Giustina G, Schalm SW, et al. Occurrence of hepatocellular carcinoma and decompensation in western European patients with cirrhosis type B. The EUROHEP Study Group on Hepatitis B Virus and Cirrhosis. Hepatology 1995;21:77–82.

29. deJohgn FE, Janssen HL, de Man RA, et al. Survival and prognostic indicators in hepatitis B surface antigen-positive cirrhosis of the liver. Gastroenterology 1992; 103:1630–5.

30. Liaw YF, Chen JJ, Chen TJ. Acute exacerbation in patients with liver cirrhosis: a clinicopathological study. Liver 1990;10:177–84.

31. Fattovich G, Pantalena M, Zagni I, et al. Effect of hepatitis B and virus infections on the natural history of compensated cirrhosis; a cohort study of 297 patients. Am J Gastroenterol 2002;97:2886–95.

32. Hui AY, Chan HL, Leung NW, et al. Survival and prognostic indicators in patients with hepatitis B virus-related cirrhosis after onset of hepatic decompensation. J Clin Gastroenterol 2002;34:569–72.

33. Das K, Datta S, Pal S, et al. Course of disease and survival after onset of decompensation in hepatitis B virus-related cirrhosis. Liver Int 2010;30:1033–42.

34. Sun LJ, Yu JW, Zhao YH, et al. Influential factors of prognosis in lamivudine treatment for patients with acute-on-chronic hepatitis B liver failure. J Gastroenterol Hepatol 2010;25:583–90.

35. Garg H, Sarin SK, Kumar M, et al. Tenofovir improves the outcome in patents with spontaneous reactivation of hepatitis B presenting as acute-on-chronic liver failure. Hepatology 2011;53:774–80.

36. Chen T, He Y, Liu X, et al. Nucleoside analogues improve the short-term and long-term prognosis of patients with hepatitis B virus-related acute-on-chronic liver failure. Clin Exp Med 2012;12:159–64.

37. Cui Y-L, Yan F, Wang Y-B, et al. Nucleoside analogue can improve the long-term prognosis of patients with hepatitis B virus infection-associated acute on chronic liver failure. Dig Dis Sci 2010;55:2373–80.

38. Eun JR, Lee HJ, Kim TN, et al. Risk assessment for the development of hepatocellular carcinoma: according to on-treatment viral response during long-term

lamivudine therapy in hepatitis B virus-related liver disease. J Hepatol 2010;53: 118–25.

39. Lin B, Pan CQ, Xie D, et al. Entecavir improves the outcome of acute-on-chronic liver failure due to the acute exacerbation of chronic hepatitis B. Hepatol Int 2013; 7:460–7.

40. Xu Q-H, Chen L-B, Xu Z, et al. The short-term efficacy of antiviral treatment in patients with acute-on-chronic hepatitis B liver failure. Zhonhua Shi Yan He Lin Chuang Bing Du Xue Za Zhi 2009;23:467–9 [in Chinese].

41. Pugh RN, Murray-Lyon IM, Dawson JL, et al. Transection of the esophagus for bleeding esophageal varices. Br J Surg 1973;60:646–9.

42. Kamat PS, Wiesner RH, Malinchoc M, et al. A model to predict survival in patients with end-stage liver disease. Hepatology 2001;33:464–70.

43. Jalan R, Saliba F, Pavesi M, et al. Development and validation of a prognostic score to predict mortality in patients with acute-on-chronic liver failure. J Hepatol 2014;61:1038–47.

44. Hadziyannis SJ. Update on Hepatitis B virus infection: focus on treatment. J Clin Translational Hepatol 2014;3:285–91.

45. Terrault NA, Bzowej NH, Chang K-M, et al. AASD guidelines for treatment of chronic hepatitis B. Hepatology 2016;63:261–83.

46. Rehermann B, Bertoletti A. Immunological aspects of antiviral therapy of chronic hepatitis B virus and hepatitis C. Virus Infections Hepatol 2014;61(2):712–21.

47. Shafritz DA, Shouval D, Sherman HI, et al. Integration of hepatitis B virus DNA into the genome of liver cells in chronic liver disease and hepatocellular carcinoma. Studies in percutaneous liver biopsies and post-mortem tissue specimens. N Eng J Med 1981;305:1067–73.

48. Brown A, Goodman Z. Hepatitis B-associated fibrosis and fibrosis/cirrhosis progression with nucleoside and nucleotide analogs. Exper Rev Gastroenterol Hepatol 2012;6:187–98.

49. Kim CH, Um SH, Seo YS, et al. Prognosis of hepatitis B-related liver cirrhosis in the era of oral nucleos(t)ide analog antiviral agents. J Gastroent Hepatol 2012; 27:1589–95.

50. Liaw YF, Sung JJ, Chow WC, et al. Lamivudine for patients with chronic hepatitis B and advanced liver disease. N Engl J Med 2004;351:1521–32.

51. Rosenau J, Bahr MJ, Tillmann HL, et al. Lamivudine and low-dose hepatitis B immune globulin for prophylaxis of hepatitis B reinfection after liver transplantation possible role of mutations in the YMDD motif prior to transplantation as a risk factor for reinfection. J Hepatol 2001;34:895–902.

52. Izzedine H, Hulot JS, Launay-Vacher V, et al. Renal safety of adefovir dipivoxil in patients with chronic hepatitis B: two double-blind, randomized, placebo-controlled studies. Kidney Int 2004;66:1153–8.

53. Papatheodoris GV, Manolakopoulos S, Dusheiko G, et al. Therapeutic strategies in the management of patients with chronic hepatitis B virus infection. Lancet Infect Dis 2008;8:167–78.

54. Papatheodoridis GV, Cholongitas E, Archimandritis AJ, et al. Current management of hepatitis B virus infection before and after liver transplantation. Liver Int 2009;29:1294–305.

55. Lok ASF, McManon BJ, Brown RS Jr, et al. Antiviral therapy for chronic hepatitis B viral infection in adults: a systemic review and meta-analysis. Hepatology 2016; 63:284–306.

56. Shim JH, Lee HC, Kim KM, et al. Efficacy of entecavir in treatment-naïve patients with hepatitis B virus-related decompensated cirrhosis. J Hepatol 2010;52(2): 176–82.

57. Liaw YF, Raptopoulou-Gigi M, Cheinquer H, et al. Efficacy and safety of entecavir versus adefovir in chronic hepatitis B patients with hepatic decompensation: a randomized, open-label study. Hepatology 2011;53(1):62–72.

58. Liaw YF, Sheen IS, Lee CM, et al. Tenofovir disoproxil fumarate (TDF), emticitabine/TDF, and entecavir in patients with decompensated chronic hepatitis B liver disease. Hepatology 2011;53(1):62–72.

59. Jang JW, Choi JY, Kim YS, et al. Long term effect of antiviral therapy on disease course after decompensation in patients with hepatitis B virus-related cirrhosis. Hepatology 2015;61:1809–20.

60. Cholongitas E, Papatheodoridis GV, Goulis J, et al. The impact of newer nucleos(t)ide analogues on patients with hepatitis B decompensated cirrhosis. Ann Gastroenterol 2015;28(1):109–17.

61. Peng C-Y, Chien R-N, Liaw Y-F. Hepatitis B virus-related decompensated liver cirrhosis: benefits of antiviral therapy. J Hepatol 2012;57:442–550.

62. DuanZ, Xin S, Zhang J, et al. 3-year follow up of acute-on-chronic liver failure (ACLF) subjects in a randomized, controlled, multicenter trial of the ELAD Bioartificial Liver Support System in 49 Chinese subjects reveals significant transplant-free survival (TFS) benefit. 61st Annual Meeting of the American Association for the Study of Liver Diseases (AASLD 2010). Boston, October 29-November 2, 2010. Abstract 1610.

63. Marzano A, Gaia S, Ghisetti V, et al. Viral load at the time of liver transplantation and risk of hepatitis B virus recurrence. Liver Transpl 2005;11:402–9.

64. Burra P, Germani G, Adam R, et al. Liver transplantation for HBV-related cirrhosis in Europe: an ELTR study on evolution and outcomes. J Hepatol 2013;58:287–96.

65. Xu X, Tu Z, Wang B, et al. A novel model of evaluating the risk of hepatitis B recurrence after liver transplantation. Liver Int 2011;31:1477–84.

66. Hu TH, Chen CL, Lin CC, et al. Section 14. Combination of entecavir plus low-dose on-demand hepatitis B immunoglobulin is effective with very low hepatitis B recurrence after liver transplantation. Transplantation 2014;97(8):S53–9.

67. Chang MS, Stiles JB, Lukose TS, et al. Adherence to hepatitis B immunoglobulin (HBIG) after liver transplantation. Transplantation 2013;96:e84–5.

68. Gane EJ, Patterson S, Strasser SI, et al. Combination of lamivudine and adefovir without hepatitis B immune globulin is safe and effective prophylaxis against hepatitis B virus recurrence in hepatitis B surface antigen-positive liver transplant candidates. Liver Transpl 2013;19:268–74.

69. Wang P, Tam N, Wang H, et al. Is hepatitis B immunoglobulin necessary in prophylaxis of hepatitis B recurrence after liver transplantation? A meta-analysis. PLoSOne 2014;9:e104480.

Hepatitis B and Risk of Non–Hepatocellular Carcinoma Malignancy

 CrossMark

Ryan M. Kwok, MD[a],*, Tram T. Tran, MD[b]

KEYWORDS

- Chronic hepatitis B • Non–hepatocellular carcinoma malignancy
- Non-Hodgkin lymphoma • Pancreatic adenocarcinoma
- Intrahepatic cholangiocarcinoma

KEY POINTS

- Hepatitis B virus (HBV) is a global public health problem with sequelae of infection, including cirrhosis and hepatocellular carcinoma (HCC); data suggest an increased risk for non-HCC malignancies and hepatitis B infection.
- The non-HCC malignancies most strongly associated with HBV infection are non-Hodgkin lymphoma, pancreatic adenocarcinoma, and intrahepatic cholangiocarcinoma.
- Mechanisms for non-HCC HBV-related carcinogenesis are thought to be related to direct mutagenesis and secondarily through chronic inflammation and fibrosis, as well as oxidative DNA damage.
- Due to the lack of clear association, screening for non-HCC malignancy in patients chronically infected with HBV is challenging; screening should involve regular, thorough history and physical examination with special attention paid to signs and symptoms suggestive of lymphoid malignancy.

INTRODUCTION

Hepatitis B virus (HBV) infection is a global public health problem with an estimated worldwide prevalence of 240 million persons.[1] The most significant sequelae of infection are cirrhosis and hepatocellular carcinoma (HCC), with HBV as the leading cause of HCC worldwide. Studies suggest 10-fold to 60-fold increased risk of HCC,

Disclosure: Dr T.T. Tran serves as an advisor/speaker, consultant, and researcher for Gilead Sciences, Bristol Myers Squibb, AbbVie, Merck, Janssenn, and Valeant. Dr R.M. Kwok has nothing to disclose.
[a] Gastroenterology Fellowship Program, Walter Reed National Military Medical Center, 8901 Wisconsin Avenue, Bethesda, MD 20889, USA; [b] Gastroenterology Fellowship Program, Cedars Sinai Medical Center, Geffen School of Medicine at University of California Los Angeles, 8900 Beverly Boulevard, Los Angeles, CA 90048, USA
* Corresponding author.
E-mail address: ryan.m.kwok.mil@mail.mil

depending on hepatitis B surface antigen (HBsAg) and hepatitis B envelope antigen (HBeAg) status, compared with the general population.[2] Although most HCC develops in HBV-related cirrhosis, infection alone is an established risk factor for noncirrhotic HCC development. The oncogenic potential of HBV cannot be understated.

Although largely considered a hepatotropic virus, HBV can also replicate in endothelial cells, macrophages/monocytes, hematopoietic precursors, stromal cells, and neuronal cells in chronic infection. This ability suggests that the presence of HBV in these cells may be associated with extrahepatic syndromes such as vasculitis, glomerulonephropathy, neuropathy, and dermatitis.[3] Thus, the potential for an association between HBV-related malignancy in these extrahepatic organs seems rational. Several studies suggest epidemiologic association between HBV and non-HCC malignancies such as non-Hodgkin lymphoma[4] (NHL), cholangiocarcinoma,[5] and pancreatic cancer.[6]

This article reviews the associations between HBV and non-HCC malignancies and offers surveillance and potential prophylactic strategies in the care of patients with chronic HBV infection (CHB).

PATHOLOGIC MECHANISMS
Hepatitis B Carcinogenesis

The carcinogenic mechanisms of hepatitis B in HCC have been well characterized. Hepatitis B directly modulates dysplasia through mutagenesis secondary to viral DNA integration into the host genome. This process increases both genomic instability and epigenomic modification through the action of the HBx viral protein. Cell death and proliferation are also modulated through overexpression of HBV-associated proteins. A secondary effect of HBV occurs through promotion of chronic inflammation and fibrosis, cell death and regeneration, and oxidative DNA damage, all of which contribute to malignant risk.[7]

Despite epidemiologic associations between HBV and non-HCC malignancies, specific mechanisms are not as well defined. Drawing on putative HCC pathways, specifically the inactivation of p53 by the HBx protein affecting repair and apoptosis, it has been suggested that similar mechanisms are at play in non-HCC malignancy.[8]

Hepatitis C: a Model for Lymphoproliferation?

There is a strong association between microbial pathogens and lymphomas through 2 primary mechanisms. Lymphotropic, oncogenic viruses such as Epstein-Barr virus, human herpesvirus 8, and human T-lymphotropic virus 1 directly infect and transform lymphoid cells. In contrast, microbes, including hepatitis C virus (HCV), *Helicobacter pylori*, *Campylobacter jejuni*, and *Chlamydophila psittaci* are associated with chronic antigenic stimulation leading to extranodal B-cell marginal zone lymphomas.[9]

A rational parallel between HBV-associated and HCV-associated NHL can be drawn by their shared hepatotropic and lymphotropic characteristics. Epidemiologic associations between HCV and B-cell NHL (B-NHL) are well described, with an ~11-fold increased risk versus healthy controls.[10] In addition, studies have shown regression of NHL after treatment of HCV, strengthening this association.[11,12] Specific pathologic mechanisms have not been described.

Theories have been proposed suggesting transformation of infected B cells through microRNA dysregulation, thus undermining tumor suppression.[13] In addition, the established role of HCV in clonal B-cell expansion seen in mixed (type II) cryoglobulinemia, increased expression of BCL2 oncogene in patients infected with HCV,[14] and disappearance of the t(14;18) translocations after antiviral treatment[15] lends pathologic clues to a virally mediated lymphomagenesis.

Evidence for Hepatitis B Lymphoproliferation

Hepatitis B DNA has been shown in both monocytes and B lymphocytes. The risk of HBV transmission by infected lymphocytes has been shown in liver transplant recipients, whereas infected monocytes have been implicated in vertical transmission.[16] Additional studies have shown the presence of HBV DNA in the bone marrow of children with leukemia.[17]

Despite the presence of HBV DNA in hematopoietic cells, the evidence for a pathologic role of HBV in lymphoid malignancy is less robust. An association between HBV and lymphoproliferation associated with mixed cryoglobulinemia was described by Levo and colleagues[18] in 1977. The serum and/or cryoprecipitate of 30 patients with essential mixed cryoglobulins (EMCs) were examined. Samples were examined for the presence of HBsAg or hepatitis B surface antibody (anti-HBs) after excluding connective tissue disease, lymphoproliferative neoplasm, or other known chronic infection. Forty-nine patients with systemic lupus erythematosus or rheumatoid arthritis were selected as controls. Hepatitis B vaccination was not initiated in the United States until 1982, suggesting that any positive serologies were attributable to chronic or prior infection. Although no P values are reported, 13 of 25 (52%) EMC serum samples were anti-HBs positive (anti-HBs+), whereas 3 of 24 (12.5%) were HBsAg positive (HBsAg+). In contrast, 12 of 49 (24%) and 0 of 49 (0%) controls were anti-HBs HBsAg+, respectively. More recent data showed massive monoclonal expression of VH1-69–expressing B cells in 2 out of 5 patients with chronic HBV with mixed cryoglobulinemia (MC). In both patients, anti-HBV therapy led to regression of the VH1-69–positive B-cells as well as the MC, suggesting that protracted HBV antigenic stimulation may contribute to these processes.[19]

Reports of remission of splenic marginal zone lymphoma after antiviral therapy for HBV also suggest a pathologic role.[20] Koot and colleagues[21] also proposed a chronic antigenic stimulation mechanism wherein HBV-host DNA integration leads to overexpression of cellular oncogenes or tumor suppressor gene downregulation. A second theory includes viral production and release of hematopoietic tumor growth factors with associated lymphocyte proliferation. Although not definitive, plausible mechanisms for the role of HBV in hematologic malignancy can be derived from these findings.

Mechanisms for Hepatitis B in Other Malignancies

Other evidence is more loosely associated and derived from the findings of HBV DNA in extrahepatic organs. For example, the shared blood supply and ducts of the liver, bile ducts, and pancreas make these organs potential targets for HBV infection and primary malignancy. This finding has been supported not only by the findings of HBsAg in pancreatic secretions and bile[22] but also by evidence of pancreatic inflammation in acute viral hepatitis.[23]

Similarly limited data exists on the pathogenic mechanism for HBV in intrahepatic cholangiocarcinoma (ICC); however, several studies have investigated the presence of HBV in pathology specimens. In these studies, a variety of HBV products were found in hepatic tissue surrounding resected ICC, including HBV DNA, the HBx gene, pre-S gene, S gene, and C gene.[24,25] Investigators have proposed a mechanism of neoplastic transformation of hepatic and cholangiocytic progenitor cells known as oval cells. It is thought that this process may give rise to both HCC and ICC.[26] Similarly, a common pathway of inflammation, cirrhosis, and carcinogenesis has been proposed because of evidence of greater inflammation and scarring in HBV ICC versus non–-HBV-related ICC.[27] In addition, similar to HCC, the HBx and p53 proteins have been shown to be present in liver tissue surrounding resected ICC.[28]

The association between chronic hepatitis B and extrahepatic malignancy, particularly NHL, warrants further study to define the possible pathogenic mechanisms.

POPULATION STUDIES
Lymphoid Malignancy

The association between HBV and non–HCC-related malignancy has been observed for more than 2 decades.[29] Similar to HCV and lymphoid malignancies,[30] several observational studies have noted a correlation between chronic HBV infection and hematologic malignancy.

In a cohort of 3888 US patients with chronic HBV, Yood and colleagues[31] found the risk of developing NHL nearly 3 times higher (adjusted hazard ratio, 2.8; 95% confidence interval, 1.16–6.75) in patients with CHB. Older, smaller studies found similar associations in Asian[32] and European cohorts.[33] Increased recognition of this association led to significantly larger population studies. In the Korean Cancer Prevention Study, Engels and colleagues[34] examined more than 53,000 HBsAg+ patients and found a hazard ratio of 1.74 (95% CI, 1.45–20.9) for NHL versus controls. An analysis of the European Prospective Investigation into Cancer and Nutrition (EPIC) cohort by Franceschi and colleagues[35] identified 1023 patients diagnosed with NHL, multiple myeloma (MM), and Hodgkin lymphoma (HL) and assessed HBV and HCV serologies. Nonsignificant associations were found between HBsAg+ patients and NHL (odds ratio [OR], 1.78; 95% CI, 0.78–4.04), MM (OR, 4.00; 95% CI, 1.00–16.0), and HL (OR, 2.0; 95% CI, 0.13–32.0). However, when the 3 malignancies were combined, a significant association was observed (OR, 2.21; 95% CI, 1.12–4.33).

Despite this, a recent study of 4345 Danish patients with HBV, Andersen and colleagues[36] found no increase in risk of NHL. One explanation for this discrepancy could be the prevalence of hepatitis B in the respective study populations.

Several studies confirm the findings of Engels and colleagues[34] that suggest the risk for HBV-related NHL seems to be highest in B-cell–subtype NHL[15,37,38] with no increased risk for T-cell NHL. Data among other lymphoid malignancies are mixed. Specifically, some studies of HL and MM have shown a positive association,[39] whereas others find no association.[34]

In summary, conflicting data exist with regard to the association between HBV and hematologic malignancies. B-cell NHL seems to have the most substantive data, and viral suppression in patients with a diagnosis of hepatitis B and NHL should be considered.

Pancreatic Cancer

Pancreatic cancer has also been shown to be associated with HBV infection. Hassan and colleagues[6] reported a 2-fold to 3-fold increased risk of developing pancreatic cancer for patients previously exposed to HBV (positive anti-HBc). A similar risk was confirmed in 2 studies examining the Taiwanese REVEAL-HBV cohort (Risk Evaluation of Viral Load Elevation and Associated Liver Disease/Cancer-Hepatitis B Virus).[40,41] Nearly 24,000 patients were followed with 23 new diagnoses of pancreatic cancer and a relative risk of developing pancreatic cancer in HBsAg+ patients of 2.4 (95% CI, 0.9–6.7). The investigators concluded that both CHB and active replication of HBV are associated with pancreatic cancer risk.

The same Danish study previously discussed by Andersen and colleagues[36] also found no association with pancreatic cancer. Additionally, others have also disputed the association between pancreatic cancer and HBV in Korea, an area that is endemic for CHB.[42]

Intrahepatic Cholangiocarcinoma

Intrahepatic cholangiocarcinoma (ICC) has also been theorized to have an association with HBV infection. However, the data are similarly heterogeneous. The findings of 3 recent meta-analyses favor an association between HBV and ICC, especially in endemic regions. Risk estimates range from 2-fold to 5-fold versus controls.[43–45]

Other Malignancy

Amin and colleagues[46] sought to examine the risk of tumors following HBV and HCV infection in a cohort of more than 120,000 Australian patients. A standardized incident ratio (SIR) of 4.4 (95% CI, 1.4–13.7) was found in cancers of unknown primary in HBV/HCV coinfected patients, whereas there was no significant association for HBV infection alone. The SIR in HBV infection for nasopharyngeal neoplasms was 3.1 (95% CI, 1.3–7.3) and 3.4 (95% CI, 1.6–7.1) in Kaposi sarcoma. The investigators noted that this association is confounded by patients' countries of birth, with all subjects with nasopharyngeal carcinoma being born in China and south east Asia, where this disease is highly prevalent. Confirming the disparate data on HBV risk in NHL, no major subgroup of NHL had an increased risk. However, the risk of subtype Burkett lymphoma was significantly increased (SIR, 11.8; 95% CI, 4.9–28.4). When the malignancy risk associated with HIV was adjusted for, Kaposi sarcoma was no longer significant, whereas Burkitt lymphoma remained significant (SIR, 12.9; 95% CI, 5.4–30.9).

HEPATITIS B VIRAL MARKERS

Factors such as serum HBV DNA level greater than 2000 IU/mL, HBsAg status, and HBeAg status are known virus-related risk factors for development of HCC.[2,47] Current data preclude drawing strong conclusions in non-HCC malignancy. Population studies use varying definitions when defining chronic hepatitis B, ranging from ICD codes to HBsAg. As such, few studies have examined the risk of non-HCC malignancy related to virus exposure (anti-HBc (anti-Hepatitis B core), anti-HBs) or replication (HBeAg, anti-HBe, HBV DNA viral load).

Non-Hodgkin Lymphoma

Most studies, including those previously discussed, use the presence of HBsAg+ when examining malignancy risk. As shown, HBsAg+ patients seem to be a risk for non-HCC malignancy, with the strongest associations with NHL. Several investigators have attempted to quantify risk associated with other serologic markers. Anti-HBc, a marker of HBV exposure, has shown mixed results regarding risk for malignancy. In an Italian cohort,[4] anti-HBc+/anti-HBs− patients were found to have a 2-fold increased risk (OR, 2.05; 95% CI, 1.24–3.37) of developing B-NHL. In the same study anti-HBs+ was found to decrease the risk for NHL with the OR in anti-HBs+/anti-HBc+ and anti-HBs+/anti-HBc− decreased to 0.89 (95% CI, 0.60–1.30) and 0.37 (95% CI, 0.20–0.73), respectively.

Wang and colleagues[38] showed a similar risk in Chinese patients in whom anti-HBc+ conferred a 1.8-fold risk (95% CI, 1.40–2.2) for NHL versus control. When examined together anti-HBs−/anti-HBc+ also had a significantly increased B-NHL risk (31% vs 17%; P<.001). This cohort also showed a protective effect of anti-HBs+ (OR, 0.6; 95% CI, 0.4–0.7). This study is the only one to assess the risk of HBeAg and anti-HBe status related to B-NHL. When examined alone, HBeAg+ and anti-HBe were found to have ORs of 1.8 (95% CI, 1.3–2.7) and 1.7 (95% CI, 1.3–2.3), respectively. The coexpression of HBsAg+ and anti-HBc+ in conjunction with HBeAg+ and anti-HBe was also associated with a significant increase compared with controls.

Pancreatic Cancer

The 2 largest studies examining the risk of pancreatic cancer also examined HBV markers other than HBsAg. The REVEAL-HBV cohort study determined a risk for HBsAg+/HBeAg+ patients of 7.3 (95% CI, 1.6–33.9) among Taiwanese patients compared with controls.[41] No data were gathered on anti-HBc status. In contrast, Hassan and colleagues[6] examined the effect of both anti-HBs and anti-HBc. HBsAg−/anti-HBc+ patients experienced a 2.5-fold increased risk (95% CI, 1.5–4.2), whereas anti-HBc+/anti-HBs− conferred a 4-fold risk (95% CI, 1.4–11.1) compared with controls. The coexpression of anti-HBc+/anti-HBs+ was associated with an OR of 2.3 (95% CI, 1.2–4.3).[6]

SURVEILLANCE

Recommendations for screening for non-HCC malignancy in chronic HBV infection are challenging primarily because of the lack of clear association. Further, the incidence of these diseases is low at baseline, making a screening/surveillance program potentially cost and resource prohibitive.

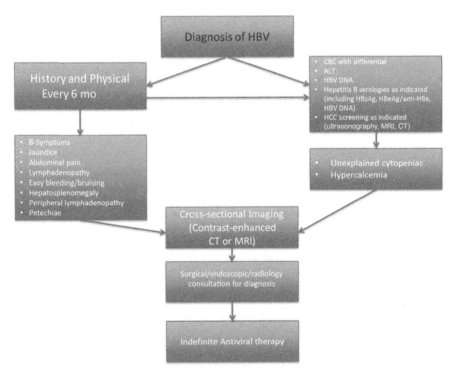

Fig. 1. Suggested approach for non-HCC malignancy surveillance in HBV patients. ALT, alanine aminotransferase; CBC, complete blood count; CT, computed tomography.

The authors recommend a regular, thorough history and physical examination at least every 6 months. Special attention should be paid to B symptoms, such as unexplained fevers, night sweats, weight loss, and fatigue. Physical examination should include evaluation for peripheral lymphadenopathy and hepatosplenomegaly. Routine laboratory work should be performed, including complete blood count, hepatic and renal function panels, and coagulation studies. In addition to regular radiographic screening as indicated for HCC, cross-sectional imaging should be considered if any concern for non-HCC malignancy exists.

See **Fig. 1** for a suggested approach to surveillance.

TREATMENT

The rationale for antiviral hepatitis B treatment in B-cell lymphoma is derived from the pathologic association between hepatitis C and B-NHL. In HCV, chronic antigenic stimulation drives lymphoproliferation and antiviral treatment is associated with tumor regression.[11,12] Accordingly, suppression of HBV viremia may lead to regression of lymphoid proliferation, mixed cryoglobulinemia,[19] and even frank malignancy.[20,21]

Treatments of certain infection-associated malignancies, such *H pylori* in mucosa-associated lymphoid tissue lymphoma, have integrated antimicrobial therapy into oncologic treatment recommendations.[48] Despite evidence showing a decreased risk in HCC associated with treated CHB,[2] no robust data exist on improved outcomes with antiviral treatment in HBV-associated, non-HCC malignancies. Accordingly, treatment of malignancy in patients with CHB should be done in a multidisciplinary fashion with an oncologist and by current standards of care. Addressing the risk of hepatitis B reactivation with immunosuppression is essential and should involve the input of a gastroenterologist/hepatologist familiar with the use of hepatitis B antiviral therapies.[49,50]

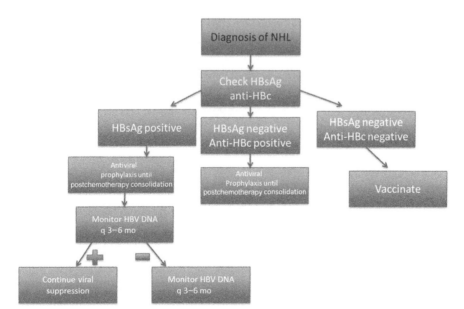

Fig. 2. Suggested screening and treatment strategy for HBV in newly diagnosed NHL. HBC, Hepatitis B core; q, every.

Cases may arise in which a patient is diagnosed with a hepatitis B–associated non-HCC malignancy and may not otherwise be a candidate for antiviral therapy (eg, immune-tolerant CHB). Expert consultation is recommended in these cases, with consideration of antiviral therapy, particularly if immunosuppression is planned. These patients should be monitored closely (eg, monthly for the first 6 months, then every 3 months) for viremia, alanine aminotransferase flares, and clinical decompensation. See **Fig. 2** for a suggested screening and treatment strategy with newly diagnosed NHL.

SUMMARY

Chronic hepatitis B infection is a known risk factor for malignancy. Unlike HCC, less is known about the risk of non-HCC malignancy. However, epidemiology and pathologic evidence suggests a strong association between NHL and CHB. Data regarding the risk of other malignancies, such as pancreatic adenocarcinoma and intrahepatic cholangiocarcinoma, are mixed. Surveillance and appropriate treatment of infection and malignancy in these patients is essential. Further study of these associations is needed and may bring new insights in the pathogenesis and treatment of these diseases.

REFERENCES

1. Ott J, Stevens G, Groeger J, et al. Global epidemiology of hepatitis B virus infection: new estimates of age specific HBsAg seroprevalence and endemicity. Vaccine 2012;30:2212–9.
2. Yang HI, Lu SN, Liaw YF, et al. Hepatitis B e antigen and the risk of hepatocellular carcinoma. N Engl J Med 2002;347:168–74.
3. Mason A, Wick M, White H, et al. Hepatitis B virus replication in diverse cell types during chronic hepatitis B virus infection. Hepatology 1993;18(4):781–4.
4. Marcucci F, Mele A, Spada E, et al. High prevalence of hepatitis B virus infection in B-cell non-Hodgkins lymphoma. Haematologica 2006;91:554–7.
5. Lee T, Lee S, Jung S, et al. Hepatitis B virus infection and intrahepatic cholangiocarcinoma in Korea: a case-control study. Am J Gastroenterol 2008;103:1716–20.
6. Hassan M, Li D, El-Deeb A, et al. Association between hepatitis B virus and pancreatic cancer. J Clin Oncol 2008;26:4557–62.
7. Guerrieri F, Belloni L, Pediconi H, et al. Molecular mechanisms of HBV-associated hepatocarcinogenesis. Semin Liver Dis 2013;33:147–56.
8. Yi HZ, Chen JJ, Cen H, et al. Association between infection of hepatitis B virus and onset risk of B-cell non-Hodgkins lymphoma: a systematic review and a meta-analysis. Med Oncol 2014;31:84.
9. Suarez F, Lortholary O, Hermine O, et al. Infection-associated lymphomas derived from marginal zone B cells: a model of antigen driven lymphoproliferation. Blood 2006;107:3034–44.
10. Gisbert J, Garcia-Buey L, Pajares J, et al. Prevalence of hepatitis C virus infection in B-cell non-Hodgkin's lymphoma.: systematic review and meta-analysis. Gastroenterology 2003;125(6):1723–32.
11. Vallisa D, Bernuzzi P, Arcaini L, et al. Role of anti-hepatitis C virus treatment in HCV-related, low-grade, B-cell, non-Hodgkin's lymphoma: a multicenter Italian experience. J Clin Oncol 2005;23(3):468–73.
12. Hermine O, Lefrere F, Bronowicki JP, et al. Regression of splenic lymphoma with villous lymphocytes after treatment of hepatitis C virus infection. N Engl J Med 2002;347(2):89–94.

13. Peveling-Oberhag J, Crisman G, Schmidt A, et al. Dysregulation of global micro-RNA expression in splenic marginal zone lymphoma and influence of chronic hepatitis C virus infection. Leukemia 2012;26:1654–62.

14. Zignengo A, Giannelli F, Marrocchi M, et al. T(14;18) translocation in chronic hepatitis C virus infection. Hepatology 2000;31:474–9.

15. Zuckerman E, Zuckerman T, Sahar D, et al. The effect of antiviral therapy on t(14;18) translocation and immunoglobulin gene rearrangement in patients with chronic hepatitis C virus infection. Blood 2001;97:1555–9.

16. Pontisso P, Vidalino L, Quarta S, et al. Biological and clinical implications of HBV infection in peripheral blood mononuclear cells. Autoimmun Rev 2008;8(1):13–7.

17. Pontisso P, Locasciulli A, Schiavon E, et al. Detection of hepatitis B virus DNA sequences in bone marrow of children with leukemia. Cancer 1987;59:292–6.

18. Levo Y, Gorevic P, Kassab H, et al. Association between hepatitis B virus and essential mixed cryoglobulinemia. N Engl J Med 1977;296:1501–4.

19. Visentini M, Pascolini S, Mitrevski M, et al. Hepatitis B virus causes mixed cryoglobulinaemia by driving clonal expansion of innate B-cells producing a VH1-69-encoded antibody. Clin Exp Rheumatol 2016;34(3 Suppl 97):28–32.

20. Christou L, Kalambokis G, Bai M, et al. Splenic marginal zone lymphoma in a patient with chronic hepatitis B. J Gastrointestin Liv Dis 2009;18(4):511–2.

21. Koot A, Visscher A, Huits R. Remission of splenic marginal zone lymphoma in a patient treated for hepatitis B: a case of HBV-associated lymphoma. Acta Clin Belg 2015;70(4):301–3.

22. Hoefs JC, Renner IG, Asklhcavai M, et al. Hepatitis B surface antigen in pancreatic and biliary secretions. Gastroenterology 1980;79:191–4.

23. Taranto D, Carrato A, Romano M, et al. Mild pancreatic damage in acute viral hepatitis. Digestion 1989;42:93–7.

24. Tao LY, He XD, Qu Q, et al. Risk factors for intrahepatic and extrahepatic cholangiocarcinoma: a case-control study in China. Liver Int 2010;30:215–21.

25. Shaib YH, El-Serag HB, Nooka AK, et al. Risk factors for intrahepatic and extrahepatic cholangiocarcinoma: a hospital-based case-control study. Am J Gastroenterol 2007;102:1016–21.

26. Zhou H, Wang H, Zhou D, et al. Hepatitis B virus-associated intrahepatic cholangiocarcinoma and hepatocellular carcinoma may hold common disease process for carcinogenesis. Eur J Cancer 2010;46:1056–61.

27. Peng NF, Li LQ, Qin X, et al. Evaluation of risk factors and clinicopathologic features for intrahepatic cholangiocarcinoma in southern China: a possible role of hepatitis B virus. Ann Surg Oncol 2011;18:1258–66.

28. Zhou YM, Cao L, Li B, et al. Expression of HBx protein in hepatitis B virus-infected intrahepatic cholangiocarcinoma. Hepatobiliary Pancreat Dis Int 2012;11:532–5.

29. Galun E, Ilan Y, Livni N, et al. Hepatitis B virus infection associated with hematopoietic tumors. Am J Pathol 1994;145(5):1001–7.

30. Engels E, Chatterjee N, Cerhan J, et al. Hepatitis C virus infection and non-Hodgkin lymphoma: results of the NCI-SEER multi-center case-control study. Int J Cancer 2004;111:76–80.

31. Yood M, Quesenberry C, Guo D, et al. Incidence of non-Hodgkin's lymphoma among individuals with chronic hepatitis B virus infection. Hepatology 2007;46:107–12.

32. Kim JH, Bang YJ, Park BJ, et al. Hepatitis B virus infection and B-cell non-Hodgkin's lymphoma in a hepatitis B endemic area: a case-control study. Jpn J Cancer Res 2002;93:471–7.

33. Cucuianu A, Patiu M, Duma M, et al. Hepatitis B and C virus infection in Romanian non-Hodgkin's lymphoma patients. Br J Haematol 1999;107:353–6.
34. Engels EA, Cho ER, Jee SH. Hepatitis B virus infection and risk of non-Hodgkin lymphoma in South Korea: a cohort study. Lancet Oncol 2010;11:827–34.
35. Francischi S, Lise M, Trepo C, et al. Infection with hepatitis B and C viruses and risk of lymphoid malignancies in the European prospective investigation into cancer and nutrition (EPIC). Cancer Epidemiol Biomarkers Prev 2011;20:208–14.
36. Andersen E, Omland L, Jepsen P, et al. Risk of all-type cancer, hepatocellular carcinoma, non-Hodgkin lymphoma and pancreatic cancer in patients infected with hepatitis B virus. J Viral Hepat 2015;22:828–34.
37. Abe S, Inoue M, Sawad N, et al. Hepatitis B and C virus infection and risk of lymphoid malignancies: a population-based cohort study (JPHC Study). Cancer Epidem 2015;39:562–6.
38. Wang F, Xu RH, Han B, et al. High incidence of hepatitis B virus in B-cell subtype non-Hodgkin lymphoma compared with other cancers. Cancer 2007;109(7): 1360–4.
39. Dalia S, Dunker K, Sokol L, et al. Hepatitis B seropositivity and risk of developing multiple myeloma or Hodgkin lymphoma: a meta-analysis of observational studies. Leuk Res 2015;39:1325–33.
40. Iloeje U, Yang H, Jen C, et al. Risk of pancreatic cancer in chronic hepatitis B virus infection: data from the REVEAL-HBV cohort study. Liver Int 2010;30(3): 423–9.
41. Yang HI, Su J, Jen CL, et al. Chronic hepatitis B infection in active replication is a risk factor for pancreatic cancer-a long term cohort study. Gastroenterology 2006; 128(4):A745.
42. de Gonzalez AB, Jee S, Engels E, et al. No association between hepatitis B and pancreatic cancer in a prospective study in Korea. J Clin Oncol 2008;27:648.
43. Li M, Li J, Li P, et al. Hepatitis B virus infection increases the risk of cholangiocarcinoma: a meta-analysis and systematic review. J Gastroenterol Hepatol 2012;27: 1561–8.
44. Zhou Y, Zhao Y, Li B, et al. Hepatitis viruses infection and risk of intrahepatic cholangiocarcinoma: evidence from a meta-analysis. BMC Cancer 2012;12:289.
45. Palmer W, Patel T. Are common factors involved in the pathogenesis of primary liver cancers? A meta-analysis of risk factors for intrahepatic cholangiocarcinoma. J Hepatol 2012;57:69–76.
46. Amin J, Dore G, O'Connell D, et al. Cancer incidence in people with hepatitis B or C infection: a large community-based linkage study. J Hepatol 2006;45:197–203.
47. Chen CJ, Yang HI, Su J, et al. Risk of hepatocellular carcinoma across a biological gradient of serum hepatitis B virus DNA level. JAMA 2006;295:65–73.
48. National Comprehensive Cancer Network. Non-Hodgkin's lymphomas (version 4.2014). Available at: http://www.nccn.org/about/nhl.pdf. Accessed February 7, 2016.
49. Perrillo RP, Gish R, Falck-Ytter YT. AGA institute technical review on prevention and treatment of hepatitis B virus reactivation during immunosuppressive drug therapy. Gastroenterology 2015;148:221–44.
50. Terrault NA, Bzowej NH, Chang KM, et al. AASLD guidelines for treatment of chronic hepatitis B. Hepatology 2016;63(1):261–83.

Hepatitis B and Hepatocellular Carcinoma

 CrossMark

Alan W. Hemming, MD, MSc, FRCSC*, Jennifer Berumen, MD,
Kristin Mekeel, MD

KEYWORDS

- Hepatocellular carcinoma • Hepatitis B • Liver transplantation • Liver resection
- Liver ablation

KEY POINTS

- Hepatocellular carcinoma is one of the leading causes of cancer death worldwide.
- Hepatitis B continues to be the most common etiologic agent worldwide in the development of hepatocellular carcinoma.
- Only early stage disease is amenable to curative therapy, such as ablation, liver resection, or liver transplantation.

INTRODUCTION

Hepatocellular carcinoma (HCC) is one of the leading causes of cancer death worldwide, and its incidence has been increasing in the last decade largely in parallel to the incidence and duration of exposure to hepatitis B and C. The global incidence of HCC is still increasing; however, the widespread implementation of hepatitis B vaccine, hepatitis B antivirals, and the introduction of direct antiviral therapies for hepatitis C virus (HCV) may have a substantial impact in reducing the incidence of HCC in the next several decades. Currently, at least in the short- to intermediate-term of the next decade, HCC remains an ongoing important issue for those patients with hepatitis B. Unfortunately, HCC has an extremely high mortality, with the annual mortality rate essentially the same as the incidence. Despite surveillance programs in patients with chronic liver disease, most tumors are diagnosed in the intermediate to advanced stage, and only palliative measures can be applied.

This report reviews the risk factors associated with the development of HCC in hepatitis B, advances in diagnosis imaging, and management of HCC.

The authors have nothing to disclose.
Division of Transplantation and Hepatobiliary Surgery, Department of Surgery, University of California, San Diego, 9300 Campus Point Drive, # 7745 La Jolla, CA 92037-1300, USA
* Corresponding author.
E-mail address: ahemming@ucsd.edu

EPIDEMIOLOGY

Liver cancer is the fifth leading cancer diagnosis in men worldwide[1] and the seventh highest cause of cancer in women, representing about 7% of the total number of cancer diagnoses. Additionally, liver cancer is the third leading cause of cancer death, after lung and stomach cancers.[2] The annual incidence of HCC is similar to the deaths per year, with most patients presenting with advanced disease with no curative options available.[1]

The overall HCC incidence increases with advancing age, with a peak at the age of 70 years.[3] In the Chinese and black African population, largely infected with hepatitis B virus (HBV), the patients are younger; in sub-Saharan Africa, it can appear, not uncommonly, in the third decade of life.[4,5]

The incidence of HCC is highest in men, with a male to female ratio of approximately 2.5 or 3 to 1.[3] The geographic distribution of HCC reflects the differences in exposure to the hepatitis viruses along with different environmental exposures. The incidence is highest in endemic areas of hepatitis B, such as East Asia and sub-Saharan Africa, with 85% of the total number of cases.[2] In most Western countries the incidence is low, with the exception of Southern Europe[6]; however, globally there is a growing incidence of the number cases of HCC, even in the West, although this is largely secondary to hepatitis C infection and more recently nonalcoholic fatty liver disease rather than hepatitis B. The introduction of vaccination against HBV in children in some endemic countries has already decreased the rate of HCC in children in those countries, and it is expected to reduce the incidence of HCC secondary to HBV in the future.[7] HCC secondary to HBV is, in theory, a preventable disease.[8]

CAUSE AND RISK FACTORS

Multiple risk factors are known to contribute to the development of HCC, the most common of those being chronic viral hepatitis (B and C), alcohol abuse, and exposure to aflatoxins; however, a small number of cases occur in people without any known risk factors.[9]

In Africa and East Asia, the most common risk factor associated with HCC is chronic HBV infection, whereas in Western countries, HCV infection is the main cause.[2] HBV continues to remain the most common etiologic agent worldwide, with 54% of cases attributed to HBV infection, 31% to HCV infection, and 15% to other causes. Cirrhosis is the largest single risk factor for the development of HCC, with 30% to 35% of cirrhotic patients going on to develop HCC at some point in their disease.[10]

HBV is a double-stranded DNA virus. The HBV genome contains 4 major open reading frames that encode for polymerase reverse transcriptase activity and replication, surface protein, and core that forms nucleocapsid as well as X protein.[11,12]

HBV-related HCC development is associated with risk factors, such as male sex, persistently high HBV DNA levels, hepatitis B e antigen (HBeAg) positivity, the presence of liver cirrhosis, older age, chronically high alanine transaminase (ALT) levels, family history of HCC or chronic infection from perinatal transmission, and coinfection with human immunodeficiency virus and/or HCV.[13–18] Males are up to 8 times more likely to develop HCC than females.[13–16] HBeAg positivity and ALT levels 45 U/L or greater are independently associated with an increased hazard ratio of developing HCC of approximately 4, whereas cirrhosis is associated with the highest increased risk of HCC development of 10 to 33 times that of patients with chronic hepatitis B that are noncirrhotic.[14,15,19] These known risk factors have been used to propose various guidelines for screening at-risk populations.

Hepatitis B Virus Genotype

Specific HBV genotypes and various mutations in genomic regions have been associated with the development of clinical manifestations, such as cirrhosis and/or HCC.[17,20] HBV has 9 genotypes (A to I) and one additional proposed genotype J.[21–23] The distribution of the different HBV genotypes is geographic and correlates with the distribution of the different ethnic populations worldwide.[23–26]

Most reports on the effect of genotype come from the Asia Pacific regions where HBV genotype B and/or C predominate. HBV genotype B is thought to be less aggressive than genotype C.[20,27,28] In general, HBV genotype C is associated with later HBe seroconversion, more severe liver disease, as well as faster progression to liver fibrosis cirrhosis and HCC development. Compared with other genotypes, genotype C has a worse progression to advanced liver disease, with a hazard ratio 2.0 to 2.3 times more than HBV genotype B or A and D, the other major HBV genotypes associated with HCC.[29] HBV genotype C reportedly has a higher tendency to induce DNA double-strand breaks and accumulate reactive oxygen species that increase the risk of chromosomal rearrangements and DNA damage, leading to the formation and development of HCC.[30]

Hepatitis B Virus Genetic Mutation

Several reports suggest that a double mutation in the basal core promoter region of the HBV genome (A1762T/G1764A) is associated with up to a 10-fold increased risk of HCC and that this is more frequent in those infected with HBV genotype C compared with genotype B.[27,31–33] In combination with other point mutations (C1653T and T1753V), these core promoter mutations are associated with an even higher risk of HCC in HBeAg-positive patients.[14,27]

Mutations in other regions of the HBV genome have also been linked with disease progression; in particular, the Pre S region is associated with the progression of chronic hepatitis and is associated with a significant increase in HCC risk.[27,34] Hepatocytes expressing assorted forms of PreS2 mutants also demonstrate increased oxidative stress due to protein retention and DNA damage while simultaneously creating genomic instability and upregulation of cell cycle progression and proliferation.[35–37] A mutation in codon 38 of the X gene was found at an increased frequency in patients with HCC and has been used as an independent risk factor for the development of HCC.[38]

Hepatitis B Virus X Protein

The involvement of viral proteins has been implicated in oncogenesis; however, their pathogenesis in HCC remains unclear because HBV infection also causes an immunologic response that in itself leads to oxidative stress and successive DNA damage to cells.[39] Integration of HBV DNA into the human genome may explain the incidence of noncirrhotic HCC.[40] This insertion can involve deletions, cis/transactivations, translocations, production of fusion transcripts, and generalized genomic instability.[41,42] However, noncirrhotic HCC with low-grade fibrosis can also be found in non–HBV-related HCC.[43,44] HBV DNA integration is present in most HBV-related HCC but can also be identified in nontumor tissue and chronic hepatitis B without HCC.[45] HBV DNA integration is generally considered to have a strong oncogenic effect in hepatocarcinogenesis.

Direct oncogenic effects of X protein and surface protein HBs have been postulated. X protein functions as a regulator in the viral life cycle, a transcriptional activator, and a stimulator in the cytoplasmic signal transduction pathways.[46] Expression of X protein was found to be present in approximately 50% to 60% of HBV-infected HCC tissues and found in the cytoplasm of both parenchymal and neoplastic cells.[47]

Integration of HBV X sequence into the host genome is a common event in HCC.[45] It has been reported that HBV X integration occurs more often in HCC than in cirrhosis.[48] Whole-genome sequencing of HCC samples has demonstrated HBV X DNA integration within or upstream of the sequence of telomerase reverse transcriptase, epigenetic regulator MLL4, and cell cycle gene *CCNE1*.[49–51] DNA integration was observed in approximately 80% of tumors but was present in only 30% of adjacent liver tissues.[51]

Hepatitis B Virus S Protein

Both PreS1 and PreS2 regions are variable and prone to genetic mutations. In animal models the insertion of PreS/S gene regions expressed high level of HBsAg, showed inflammation and appearance of preneoplastic lesions, and finally led to HCC in most animals,[52] and suggests a direct oncogenic effect. Gene expression profile of mice with this insertion showed differentially expressed genes involved in various regulatory functions such as apoptosis, cell cycle, NF-κB signal transduction pathway, and inflammatory response.[53]

A recent study reported that patients with HCC with occult hepatitis B had HBV DNA integration in approximately 75% of cases. The inserted viral genes were mainly X and PreS/S, followed by C and polymerase sequences.[54] Additionally, in a prospective 12-year study in patients with chronic hepatitis C with occult hepatitis B infection, X integration was associated with HCC development in the absence of cirrhosis.[55]

SURVEILLANCE

Surveillance is only cost-effective in populations with a high prevalence of HCC. Guidelines for surveillance include patients who have a 1.5% chance of developing HCC or higher. The HBV-infected patients who meet these criteria include Asian men older than 40 years, Asian women older than 50 years, patients with HBV and cirrhosis, patients with a family history of HCC, and Africans.[56]

Patients meeting criteria includes both cirrhotic patients with HBV and in some cases noncirrhotic patients with chronic HBV infection. Most studies of surveillance for HCC in chronic liver disease have been developed in Asian countries with a high incidence of HBV. The only prospective study comparing groups of screened versus nonscreened patients was reported from China exclusively in patients with HBV infection.[57] In that study, the mortality related to HCC was lower in patients under HCC surveillance. Other retrospective studies conducted in Europe and the United States have also demonstrated a better prognosis in patients diagnosed at an earlier stage in surveillance programs.[58–60] American, European, and Asian guidelines recommended that patients at high risk of developing HCC should be entered into surveillance programs, with current recommendations suggesting that ultrasound be performed every 6 months.[56,61,62] Ultrasound is universally the modality of choice for screening, as it remains cost-effective with little if any risk to patients.[63] Ultrasound is, however, very operator dependent; additionally, many cirrhotic patients have liver characteristics that make ultrasound surveillance difficult. Lesions that are less than a centimeter are followed up in 3 months with repeat ultrasound. If the lesion remains stable in size, then ultrasound is repeated every 3 months; however, if there is evidence of growth, further imaging should be performed. Lesions greater than 1 cm should undergo further investigation with either computed tomography (CT) or MRI. Ultrasound alone has a reported sensitivity of 58% to 89% and a specificity of more than 90%.[64,65]

Ultrasound does not subject the patients to any contrast, which may be a concern for many patients with underlying cirrhosis and concomitant renal disease. The accuracy of ultrasound may be affected by underlying nodular cirrhosis, however, which is present in most of these patients with chronically diseased liver.[66,67]

Alpha-fetoprotein (AFP) has been suggested in combination with ultrasound as the method of choice for screening the patients at high risk for developing HCC; however, the American Association for the Study of Liver Disease (AASLD) has not included AFP in their recommendations because of the lack of sensitivity and specificity provided by AFP.[68] The sensitivity of AFP alone has been reported to range from 25% to 65% for detecting HCC as a screening tool and continues to be debated in its combination use with ultrasound.[69] AFP levels of greater than 1000 have been shown to be a poor prognostic factor in both liver resection and liver transplantation (LT) and is associated with a high risk of disease recurrence.[70,71]

DIAGNOSIS OF HEPATOCELLULAR CARCINOMA

There are a variety of imaging and diagnostic techniques that can be used to help make the diagnosis of HCC in patients who are found to have nodules on screening or other initial presentation.

CT scanning remains the workhorse in diagnosing HCC. The sensitivity of CT is reported at 81% as compared with 91% with MRI in a meta-analysis of 15 comparative studies between MRI and multi-detector CT. The specificity of CT was 93% compared with 95% with MRI. However, CT is a more rapid and less operator-dependent imaging technique. Arterial enhancement and portal venous phase washout in a lesion in a cirrhotic liver suggests the diagnosis of HCC (**Fig. 1**).[72]

CT imaging does place patients at some risk for contrast-induced nephropathy, and its use may be limited in patients with decreased renal function. Serious nephrotoxicity is, however, a rare event.[73]

The presence of typical imaging features in a lesion greater than 1 cm with arterial enhancement and portal phase washout on either CT or MRI in a cirrhotic liver is pathognomonic for HCC and does not mandate biopsy for confirmation. In fact, in many cases biopsy is contraindicated and should be avoided. In cases when diagnosis is uncertain or when it will change management, biopsy remains a useful tool.

In the cirrhotic liver, multiple nodules may be observed that may not meet the full diagnostic criteria for HCC. The American College of Radiology has developed a new classification to assign risk to these nodules. Liver Imaging-Reporting and Data

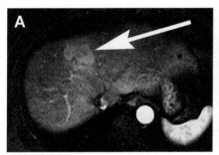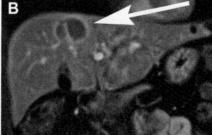

Fig. 1. MRI demonstrating arterial phase enhancement (*A*) and portal venous phase washout (*B*). The arrows indicate the lesion in segment 4a/8 of the liver, and this patient's findings on imaging are pathognomonic of HCC.

System (LI-RADS) assigns imaging findings to one of 5 categories, allowing stratification of individual observations according to the level of concern for HCC. LR-1 (LI-RADS) is an observation definitively benign and LR-5 is definitively HCC. The intermediate stages correlates with probably benign (LR-2), intermediate possibility of being HCC (LR-3), and probably HCC (LR-4) according to radiologic features, lesion size, and contrast-enhanced behavior.[74] A consensus is necessary between different organizations in order to optimize reporting of CT and MRI features in the patients at risk for HCC and to obtain consensus on the role of further investigation in lesions categorized as less than LI-RADS 5.[75]

STAGING

The main predictors of prognosis in patients with HCC are underlying liver function, tumor burden (size, number of HCC nodules, and vascular invasion), serum AFP level, and performance status. There is no universally adopted staging system for HCC. The American Joint Committee on Cancer has applied the TNM classification of malignant tumors to HCC for oncology. The United Network for Organ Sharing, the organ allocation administration in the United States, allocates donors' organs for LT for the transplantation of HCC based on a modified TNM classification in which T1 tumors (<2 cm) are not eligible for Model for End-Stage Liver Disease (MELD) exception points; T2 tumors within the Milan Criteria[76] receive exception points to allow timely transplantation, and select T3 tumors can be downstaged and potentially be eligible for subsequent transplantation. Neither staging system incorporates an assessment of hepatocellular reserve, which is critical in determining options for treatment in HCC. The first staging system specifically designed for HCC was the Okuda classification[77]; but other staging systems have been subsequently described: Cancer of the Liver Italian Program,[78] French classification,[79] Barcelona clinic liver cancer (BCLC) classification,[80] Chinese University Prognosis Index,[81] the Japan Integrated Staging,[82] among others. Each system has its proponents, and there is no consensus on a single system.

Currently, the AASLD and the European Association for the Study of Liver (EASL) endorse the use of the BCLC classification and recommend the use of this staging system for prognosis prediction and treatment.[56,62] The BCLC classification divides patients with HCC into 5 stages (0, A, B, C, D) according to preestablished prognostic factors: size and number of nodules, vascular invasion, performance status, and Child-Pugh stage. The 5 stages are as follows: 0 very early stage, A early, B intermediate, C advanced, and D terminal. Early stage patients are selected for potential curative treatments that include percutaneous ablation, surgical resection, or LT. Intermediate stage patients may be treated with chemoembolization or liver-directed therapy, whereas advanced stages may be treated with systemic therapy, such as sorafenib. Terminal patients are recommended to have only the best supportive care. The BCLC approach is put forth as a guideline only, and care of patients should remain individualized because some intermediate patients may in fact be eligible for curative options, such as transplantation.

TREATMENT

Management of patients with HCC must take into account multiple factors, including liver function, size and number of nodules, tumor extension, age, and medical comorbidities. Treatments can be divided into surgical treatment (resection or transplantation), percutaneous ablation (ethanol, microwave, radiofrequency, cryoablation and irreversible electroporation), chemoembolization, radio embolization, and systemic treatment. The choice of surgical versus, nonsurgical therapy can be complex and in each case is individualized based on many factors; team management by a multi-disciplinary group is mandatory to obtain good results in terms of survival, treatment morbidity and mortality, and recurrence. Decisions are best made in conjunction with a multidisciplinary HCC team including surgeon, hepatologist, oncologist, radiologist, and interventional radiologist. The choice of therapy in each case is individualized based on many factors; team management is mandatory to obtain good results in terms of survival, treatment morbidity and mortality, and recurrence.

Surgery

Surgical resection should be considered in any patients with HCC. Unfortunately, most patients present with unresectable disease whether due to tumor burden or poor underlying liver function. Patients who can be resected have an estimated 5-year survival of 50% to 60%, though disease-free survival is considerably less.[83] Liver resection in cirrhotic patients should have an expected perioperative mortality of less than 5%. Anatomic resection aiming at a 2-cm margin provides optimal results; however, many patients cannot tolerate extensive resections, and a balance between margin and preserving liver function must be chosen (**Fig. 2**). Selection of patients for hepatic resection involves assessment of liver function, using MELD score, Child-Pugh class, or more sophisticated measurements of hepatocellular reserve, such as the measurement of indocyanine green clearance.[84] Patients with suspected portal hypertension can be assessed by measuring the hepatic venous pressure gradient (HVPG).[85] Portal hypertension is an extremely poor prognosticator for resection, and careful assessment is required before embarking on resection. Patients with platelet counts less than 100,000/mL, splenomegaly, esophageal varices, and/or elevated HVPG are poor resection candidates.[85]

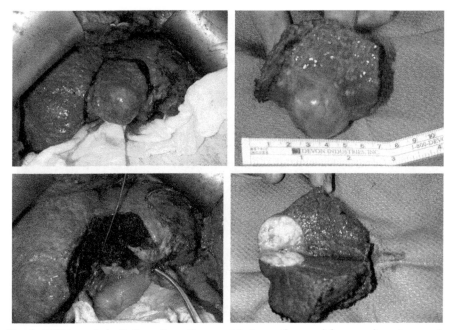

Fig. 2. HCC in a cirrhotic liver. Resection must balance the need for an adequate margin versus the need for preservation of hepatic function.

In patients with preserved function and minimal or no portal hypertension, resection can be undertaken. Tumor characteristics, such as size, multi-nodularity, and vascular invasion, are well-known predictors of recurrence and survival. HCC has a predilection for venous invasion (**Fig. 3**). Select patients with macrovascular invasion of the main, right, or left portal veins can be resected (**Fig. 4**), though results are, not surprisingly, worse than without vascular invasion. Characteristically, microscopic vascular invasion is related to tumor size and involves 20% of 2-cm tumors, 30% to 60% of tumors of 2 to 5 cm, and up to 60% to 90% of tumors more than 5 cm.[86]

Liver Transplantation

Initial results with LT for large HCC were dismal, and transplantation for HCC in the early 1990s was controversial. Mazzaferro and colleagues[76] described the Milan criteria in 1996. The Milan criteria are based on tumor size and number, allowing a solitary tumor less than 5 cm in diameter or up to 3 tumors, none of which is larger than 3 cm in diameter, with the absence of extrahepatic or vascular invasion. With the Mazzaferro and colleagues' report, LT became a viable option for curative treatment. In theory LT not only removes the tumor but also replaces the poorly functioning cirrhotic liver. Since the initial Milan study, numerous reports have validated the excellent results of liver LT for early HCC.[71,87–91] More recent studies have demonstrated that LT may represent a better option for curative treatment than resection in patients who survive to transplantation; however, given the shortage of donor livers and the high mortality and dropout rate while on the waitlist, it is not feasible to have all patients with HCC considered for transplantation.[83] The role of pretransplant chemoembolization is generally thought to be useful, largely as a bridge to transplant, maintaining control of the tumor while awaiting an organ; however, no randomized

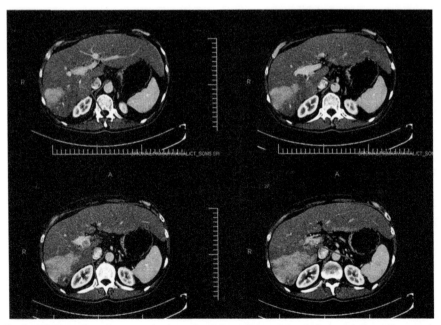

Fig. 3. HCC invading the posterior branch of the right portal vein (*arrows*). Resection can be performed in select cases even with extension to the side of the liver ipsilateral to the tumor.

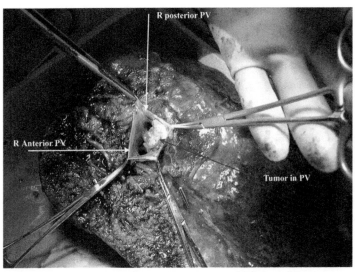

Fig. 4. The resection specimen from **Fig. 3** demonstrating tumor extruding from the posterior branch of the right portal vein to the main right portal vein. PV, portal vein; R, right.

trials assessing the utility of pretransplant chemoembolization have been completed to date.

With the initial excellent results with transplantation reported for HCC, expanded eligibility criteria beyond the Milan criteria have been proposed in order to offer life-saving transplantation to a further group of patients who might benefit. The University of California, San Francisco (UCSF) criteria is the most commonly used extension to the Milan criteria and has been applied in clinical practice.[71] Patients who underwent transplantation with a single tumor less 6.5 cm in diameter, or 2 to 3 tumors each less than 4.5 cm in diameter, with a total tumor diameter less than 8.0 cm had a similar survival to patients who underwent transplantation within the Milan criteria. Subsequent studies have validated the favorable results with the expanded criteria.[92,93] Other expanded criteria have been proposed, including another report from Mazzaferro and colleagues,[90] using the up to 7 criteria: the sum of the number of tumor nodules and the diameter of the largest nodule (in centimeters) being less than 7. These results have been validated in independent cohorts.[94,95] What has been clear is that as the criteria expand further, the rates of vascular invasion and the subsequent HCC recurrence rate begins to increase. What an acceptable level of recurrence is has yet to be defined. The international consensus conference for LT for HCC recommendations was to consider LT in patients with HCC inside the Milan criteria with only a modest expansion of the number of potential candidates outside of the Milan criteria.[96]

Downstaging

The role of downstaging in patients with HCC exceeding the Milan criteria using locoregional therapies has also been addressed: Ablation, transarterial chemoembolization (TACE), or transarterial radioembolization can be used to decrease tumor size or number to within the Milan criteria and allow transplantation. Several reports suggest successful results with this strategy, achieving 5-year survival similar to that of patients with HCC who meet the Milan criteria without requiring downstaging.[97,98] Downstaging is accompanied by an observation time during which extension of disease precludes transplantation. Downstaging in this context is likely selecting out the less biologically aggressive tumors that will respond well to transplantation. The exact starting point (UCSF, up to 7, and so forth) from which downstaging is allowed remains a focus of controversy as does the recommended observation time. The recommendation of the HCC Consensus Conference was that LT may be considered after successful downstaging, therapy, and using criteria, including size and number of viable tumor.[96]

Interventional Radiology Treatment

Most patients who present with HCC are not candidates for either surgical resection or transplantation. In these patients, liver-directed therapy offers options to control tumor growth and extend survival. In patients who are transplant candidates, liver-directed therapy may also act as a bridge to transplantation.

Percutaneous ethanol injection (PEI) was widely used until approximately 2000,[99] but it has been largely replaced with more effective energy devices. PEI may still have a role in lesions that are in close proximity to major vascular structures that preclude effective thermal approaches.

Radiofrequency ablation (RFA) has been shown to be more effective than alcohol ablation and demonstrates better control of disease.[100] RFA and, more recently, microwave ablation creates a larger area of necrosis, including a zone of necrosis or margin that extends beyond the border of the tumor. RFA creates a complete zone of necrosis with a predictable diameter. This zone can, however, be affected by nearby larger-sized vessels that act as effective heat sinks and make the area in proximity to the vascular structures resistant to heating. The heat-sink effect and the presence of nontreated microsatellites are limitations of RFA and microwaves. Ultrasound visualization of the nodule within liver parenchyma and the risk of damage to nearby organs may also limit the application of ablation.

RFA is effective in lesions less than 3 cm; however, recurrence rates increase quickly as the tumor diameter increases to greater than 3 cm. Several studies have shown that RFA is equivalent to resection in cirrhotic patients with tumors 3 cm or less. Although there is a higher local recurrence rate with ablation, there is less associated procedural mortality. In the last BCLC protocol review, RFA was considered as the first-line therapy for HCCs less than 2 cm in patients who were not candidates for LT. Microwave ablation is emerging as an alternative to RFA with several advantages. It is able to induce greater intratumoral temperature and bigger ablation area in less time than RFA, which theoretically results in less heat-sink effects. Although there are no direct comparisons of microwave with RFA, the authors have largely switched over to microwave as their energy ablation technique of choice. Irreversible electroporation (IRE) is a newly introduced technique with less clinical data available. In theory it is not affected by the heat-sink effect and does not damage adjacent structures. The exact role of IRE remains to be ascertained.[101]

TACE has been established by a meta-analysis of randomized controlled trials (RCTs) as the standard of care for nonsurgical patients with intermediate stage HCC that consist of large or multinodular noninvasive HCC isolated to the liver and with preserved liver function.[102] There are also several large series of patients with early stage single nodule, stage A HCC treated by TACE reported with good results.[103,104] Often TACE will be used as primary therapy when RFA or microwaves cannot be technically performed. In this setting, complete responses can be seen; from these observations, it has been suggested that TACE be included as an alternative curative-intent therapy in selected patients.[105]

The TACE technique remains controversial. Bland embolization or simple chemoinfusion has evolved to combined techniques of intra-arterial chemotherapy followed by induction of ischemia with intra-arterial embolic materials (TACE).

Conventional TACE involves the selective injection of a chemotherapeutic agent, such as doxorubicin emulsified in a viscous carrier (lipiodol), followed by embolic material into the feeding arteries of the tumor. This treatment has been the usual way to perform TACE and has level 1 evidence of its efficacy and remains acceptable with widespread use in Eastern countries.[102]

An alternative technique to TACE that has become popular in Western clinical practice is the use of drug-eluting beads TACE (DEB-TACE). Microspheres loaded with chemotherapeutic agents are delivered into the tumor with induction of flow cessation, which allows the delivery of large amounts of drugs to the tumor and high-dose local chemotherapy with minimal systemic effects. The Precision V trial, a prospective multi-institutional RCT, demonstrated significantly better tolerance compared with conventional TACE but demonstrated improved response only in advanced disease (Child-Pugh B).[106] More recent cohort studies and RCTs favor DEB-TACE over conventional TACE; however, which technique is best remains controversial based on the evidence to date. Ablative therapies and chemoembolization form the interventional treatments recommended by BCLC staging and treatment strategy, with simplicity as one of its known advantages. However, the huge variability of patients with HCC makes it necessary to create a tailored approach to each patient.[107] Often TACE, RFA, and transplantation are used as part of management in the same patient. The appropriate choice of therapy and development of a treatment plan requires multidisciplinary management teams and is best performed as a team approach.

Sorafenib

Sorafenib is a small molecule tyrosine kinase inhibitor that inhibits tumor-cell proliferation and tumor angiogenesis. The initial phase II and phase III studies demonstrated better survival in patients with advanced disease treated with sorafenib with an increase in the median survival from 7.9 months in the placebo group to 10.7 months in those patients receiving sorafenib. Sorafenib showed a significant benefit in time to progression, but objective responses rates were low.[108] These results were corroborated in a second phase III study conducted in Asia.[109] Sorafenib was approved for patients with preserved liver function and advanced disease not amenable to other therapies. In this group of patients, sorafenib was thought to have an acceptable safety profile with manageable adverse events. The initial results were promising despite showing only a 3-month improvement in survival because it was the first study that demonstrated that a systemic therapy had any beneficial effect in patients with HCC. Two subsequent trials, the Sorafenib or Placebo in Combination with TACE for Intermediate-Stage HCC (SPACE) and the Sorafenib or Placebo after Resection or Ablation to Prevent Recurrence of HCC (STORM), have failed to demonstrate the efficacy of sorafenib as an adjuvant modality in combination with liver-directed therapy.[110,111] Multiple novel targeted agents are under investigation in the hopes of identifying effective therapy; however, to date none have shown an improved effect over sorafenib. Both the AASLD and EASL recommend the use of sorafenib in patients with advanced-stage HCC and preserved liver function.

SUMMARY

HCC has a high incidence in patients with hepatitis B and liver cirrhosis and is currently the leading cause of death in this group of patients. HCC is expected to decrease in incidence in the coming decades because of better management of patients infected with HBV, vaccination against hepatitis B, and the extended use of antiviral drugs. In the short- to medium-term, however, HCC will remain an issue for patients with hepatitis B. Screening patient populations at risk for HCC has been shown to reduce mortality, with only patients with early stage disease being amenable to curative management, whether that is liver resection, local ablation, or LT. Improvements in imaging techniques allow diagnosis without biopsy or histologic confirmation in a high percentage of patients. Management of underlying liver disease, specialized imaging, interventional radiology, radiation oncology, and surgery may all be required. The treatment of patients with HCC is complex, with management in a multidisciplinary team setting optimal.

REFERENCES

1. Jemal A, Bray F, Center MM, et al. Global cancer statistics. CA Cancer J Clin 2011;61(2):69–90.
2. Parkin DM, Bray F, Ferlay J, et al. Global cancer statistics, 2002. CA Cancer J Clin 2005;55(2):74–108.
3. El-Serag HB, Mason AC. Rising incidence of hepatocellular carcinoma in the United States. N Engl J Med 1999;340(10):745–50.
4. Tsukuma H, Hiyama T, Tanaka S, et al. Risk factors for hepatocellular carcinoma among patients with chronic liver disease. N Engl J Med 1993;328(25): 1797–801.
5. Prates MD, Torres FO. A cancer survey in Lourenco Marques, Portuguese East Africa. J Natl Cancer Inst 1965;35(5):729–57.
6. Bosetti C, Levi F, Boffetta P, et al. Trends in mortality from hepatocellular carcinoma in Europe, 1980-2004. Hepatology 2008;48(1):137–45.
7. Franceschi S, Raza SA. Epidemiology and prevention of hepatocellular carcinoma. Cancer Lett 2009;286(1):5–8.
8. Chang MH. Cancer prevention by vaccination against hepatitis B. Recent Results Cancer Res 2009;181:85–94.
9. Bralet MP, Regimbeau JM, Pineau P, et al. Hepatocellular carcinoma occurring in nonfibrotic liver: epidemiologic and histopathologic analysis of 80 French cases. Hepatology 2000;32(2):200–4.
10. Sangiovanni A, Prati GM, Fasani P, et al. The natural history of compensated cirrhosis due to hepatitis C virus: a 17-year cohort study of 214 patients. Hepatology 2006;43(6):1303–10.
11. Shlomai A, de Jong YP, Rice CM. Virus associated malignancies: the role of viral hepatitis in hepatocellular carcinoma. Semin Cancer Biol 2014;26:78–88.
12. Dandri M, Locarnini S. New insight in the pathobiology of hepatitis B virus infection. Gut 2012;61(Suppl 1):i6–17.
13. Bosch FX, Ribes J, Diaz M, et al. Primary liver cancer: worldwide incidence and trends. Gastroenterology 2004;127(5 Suppl 1):S5–16.
14. Chen CJ, Yang HI, Su J, et al. Risk of hepatocellular carcinoma across a biological gradient of serum hepatitis B virus DNA level. JAMA 2006;295(1):65–73.
15. Kim GA, Lee HC, Kim MJ, et al. Incidence of hepatocellular carcinoma after HBsAg seroclearance in chronic hepatitis B patients: a need for surveillance. J Hepatol 2015;62(5):1092–9.
16. Li Y, Zhang Z, Shi J, et al. Risk factors for naturally-occurring early-onset hepatocellular carcinoma in patients with HBV-associated liver cirrhosis in China. Int J Clin Exp Med 2015;8(1):1205–12.

17. Pollack HJ, Kwon SC, Wang SH, et al. Chronic hepatitis B and liver cancer risks among Asian immigrants in New York City: results from a large, community-based screening, evaluation, and treatment program. Cancer Epidemiol Biomarkers Prev 2014;23(11):2229–39.
18. Shimakawa Y, Lemoine M, Bottomley C, et al. Birth order and risk of hepatocellular carcinoma in chronic carriers of hepatitis B virus: a case-control study in the Gambia. Liver Int 2015;35(10):2318–26.
19. van Bommel F, Berg T. Treatment of HBV related cirrhosis. Liver Int 2013; 33(Suppl 1):176–81.
20. Chan HL, Wong ML, Hui AY, et al. Hepatitis B virus genotype C takes a more aggressive disease course than hepatitis B virus genotype B in hepatitis B e antigen-positive patients. J Clin Microbiol 2003;41(3):1277–9.
21. Kramvis A. Genotypes and genetic variability of hepatitis B virus. Intervirology 2014;57(3–4):141–50.
22. Pourkarim MR, Amini-Bavil-Olyaee S, Kurbanov F, et al. Molecular identification of hepatitis B virus genotypes/subgenotypes: revised classification hurdles and updated resolutions. World J Gastroenterol 2014;20(23):7152–68.
23. Kurbanov F, Tanaka Y, Mizokami M. Geographical and genetic diversity of the human hepatitis B virus. Hepatol Res 2010;40(1):14–30.
24. Kramvis A, Kew M, Francois G. Hepatitis B virus genotypes. Vaccine 2005; 23(19):2409–23.
25. Thedja MD, Muljono DH, Nurainy N, et al. Ethnogeographical structure of hepatitis B virus genotype distribution in Indonesia and discovery of a new subgenotype, B9. Arch Virol 2011;156(5):855–68.
26. Westland C, Delaney W, Yang H, et al. Hepatitis B virus genotypes and virologic response in 694 patients in phase III studies of adefovir dipivoxil1. Gastroenterology 2003;125(1):107–16.
27. Liu S, Zhang H, Gu C, et al. Associations between hepatitis B virus mutations and the risk of hepatocellular carcinoma: a meta-analysis. J Natl Cancer Inst 2009;101(15):1066–82.
28. Orito E, Mizokami M. Hepatitis B virus genotypes and hepatocellular carcinoma in Japan. Intervirology 2003;46(6):408–12.
29. Wong GL, Chan HL, Yiu KK, et al. Meta-analysis: the association of hepatitis B virus genotypes and hepatocellular carcinoma. Aliment Pharmacol Ther 2013; 37(5):517–26.
30. Datta S, Roychoudhury S, Ghosh A, et al. Distinct distribution pattern of hepatitis B virus genotype C and D in liver tissue and serum of dual genotype infected liver cirrhosis and hepatocellular carcinoma patients. PLoS One 2014;9(7): e102573.
31. Constantinescu I, Dinu AA, Boscaiu V, et al. Hepatitis B virus core promoter mutations in patients with chronic hepatitis B and hepatocellular carcinoma in Bucharest, Romania. Hepat Mon 2014;14(10):e22072.
32. Kao JH, Chen PJ, Lai MY, et al. Basal core promoter mutations of hepatitis B virus increase the risk of hepatocellular carcinoma in hepatitis B carriers. Gastroenterology 2003;124(2):327–34.
33. Yotsuyanagi H, Hino K, Tomita E, et al. Precore and core promoter mutations, hepatitis B virus DNA levels and progressive liver injury in chronic hepatitis B. J Hepatol 2002;37(3):355–63.
34. Oba U, Koga Y, Hoshina T, et al. An adolescent female having hepatocellular carcinoma associated with hepatitis B virus genotype H with a deletion mutation in the pre-S2 region. J Infect Chemother 2015;21(4):302–4.

35. Hsieh YH, Chang YY, Su IJ, et al. Hepatitis B virus pre-S2 mutant large surface protein inhibits DNA double-strand break repair and leads to genome instability in hepatocarcinogenesis. J Pathol 2015;236(3):337–47.

36. Su IJ, Wang LH, Hsieh WC, et al. The emerging role of hepatitis B virus pre-S2 deletion mutant proteins in HBV tumorigenesis. J Biomed Sci 2014;21:98.

37. Wang HC, Huang W, Lai MD, et al. Hepatitis B virus pre-S mutants, endoplasmic reticulum stress and hepatocarcinogenesis. Cancer Sci 2006;97(8):683–8.

38. Muroyama R, Kato N, Yoshida H, et al. Nucleotide change of codon 38 in the X gene of hepatitis B virus genotype C is associated with an increased risk of hepatocellular carcinoma. J Hepatol 2006;45(6):805–12.

39. Higgs MR, Chouteau P, Lerat H. 'Liver let die': oxidative DNA damage and hepatotropic viruses. J Gen Virol 2014;95(Pt 5):991–1004.

40. Nault JC. Pathogenesis of hepatocellular carcinoma according to aetiology. Best Pract Res Clin Gastroenterol 2014;28(5):937–47.

41. Bonilla Guerrero R, Roberts LR. The role of hepatitis B virus integrations in the pathogenesis of human hepatocellular carcinoma. J Hepatol 2005;42(5): 760–77.

42. Ringelhan M, O'Connor T, Protzer U, et al. The direct and indirect roles of HBV in liver cancer: prospective markers for HCC screening and potential therapeutic targets. J Pathol 2015;235(2):355–67.

43. Albeldawi M, Soliman M, Lopez R, et al. Hepatitis C virus-associated primary hepatocellular carcinoma in non-cirrhotic patients. Dig Dis Sci 2012;57(12): 3265–70.

44. Kawada N, Imanaka K, Kawaguchi T, et al. Hepatocellular carcinoma arising from non-cirrhotic nonalcoholic steatohepatitis. J Gastroenterol 2009;44(12): 1190–4.

45. Tsai WL, Chung RT. Viral hepatocarcinogenesis. Oncogene 2010;29(16): 2309–24.

46. Bouchard MJ, Schneider RJ. The enigmatic X gene of hepatitis B virus. J Virol 2004;78(23):12725–34.

47. Su Q, Schroder CH, Hofmann WJ, et al. Expression of hepatitis B virus X protein in HBV-infected human livers and hepatocellular carcinomas. Hepatology 1998; 27(4):1109–20.

48. Peng Z, Zhang Y, Gu W, et al. Integration of the hepatitis B virus X fragment in hepatocellular carcinoma and its effects on the expression of multiple molecules: a key to the cell cycle and apoptosis. Int J Oncol 2005;26(2):467–73.

49. Fujimoto A, Totoki Y, Abe T, et al. Whole-genome sequencing of liver cancers identifies etiological influences on mutation patterns and recurrent mutations in chromatin regulators. Nat Genet 2012;44(7):760–4.

50. Jiang Z, Jhunjhunwala S, Liu J, et al. The effects of hepatitis B virus integration into the genomes of hepatocellular carcinoma patients. Genome Res 2012; 22(4):593–601.

51. Sung WK, Zheng H, Li S, et al. Genome-wide survey of recurrent HBV integration in hepatocellular carcinoma. Nat Genet 2012;44(7):765–9.

52. Chisari FV, Klopchin K, Moriyama T, et al. Molecular pathogenesis of hepatocellular carcinoma in hepatitis B virus transgenic mice. Cell 1989;59(6):1145–56.

53. Barone M, Spano D, D'Apolito M, et al. Gene expression analysis in HBV transgenic mouse liver: a model to study early events related to hepatocarcinogenesis. Mol Med 2006;12(4–6):115–23.

54. Saitta C, Tripodi G, Barbera A, et al. Hepatitis B virus (HBV) DNA integration in patients with occult HBV infection and hepatocellular carcinoma. Liver Int 2015; 35(10):2311–7.

55. Toyoda H, Kumada T, Kaneoka Y, et al. Impact of hepatitis B virus (HBV) X gene integration in liver tissue on hepatocellular carcinoma development in serologically HBV-negative chronic hepatitis C patients. J Hepatol 2008;48(1):43–50.

56. Bruix J, Sherman M, American Association for the Study of Liver Diseases. Management of hepatocellular carcinoma: an update. Hepatology 2011;53(3): 1020–2.

57. Zhang BH, Yang BH, Tang ZY. Randomized controlled trial of screening for hepatocellular carcinoma. J Cancer Res Clin Oncol 2004;130(7):417–22.

58. Sangiovanni A, Del Ninno E, Fasani P, et al. Increased survival of cirrhotic patients with a hepatocellular carcinoma detected during surveillance. Gastroenterology 2004;126(4):1005–14.

59. Trevisani F, De Notariis S, Rapaccini G, et al. Semiannual and annual surveillance of cirrhotic patients for hepatocellular carcinoma: effects on cancer stage and patient survival (Italian experience). Am J Gastroenterol 2002;97(3):734–44.

60. Pascual S, Irurzun J, Zapater P, et al. Usefulness of surveillance programmes for early diagnosis of hepatocellular carcinoma in clinical practice. Liver Int 2008; 28(5):682–9.

61. Poon D, Anderson BO, Chen LT, et al. Management of hepatocellular carcinoma in Asia: consensus statement from the Asian Oncology Summit 2009. Lancet Oncol 2009;10(11):1111–8.

62. European Association For The Study Of The Liver, European Organisation For Research And Treatment Of Cancer. EASL-EORTC clinical practice guidelines: management of hepatocellular carcinoma. J Hepatol 2012;56(4):908–43.

63. Hennedige T, Venkatesh SK. Imaging of hepatocellular carcinoma: diagnosis, staging and treatment monitoring. Cancer Imaging 2013;12:530–47.

64. Bolondi L. Screening tests for hepatocellular carcinoma. Hepatology 2003; 37(6):1493 [author reply: 1493].

65. Singal A, Volk ML, Waljee A, et al. Meta-analysis: surveillance with ultrasound for early-stage hepatocellular carcinoma in patients with cirrhosis. Aliment Pharmacol Ther 2009;30(1):37–47.

66. Montes Ramirez ML, Miro JM, Quereda C, et al. Incidence of hepatocellular carcinoma in HIV-infected patients with cirrhosis: a prospective study. J Acquir Immune Defic Syndr 2014;65(1):82–6.

67. Willatt JM, Hussain HK, Adusumilli S, et al. MR imaging of hepatocellular carcinoma in the cirrhotic liver: challenges and controversies. Radiology 2008; 247(2):311–30.

68. Thompson Coon J, Rogers G, Hewson P, et al. Surveillance of cirrhosis for hepatocellular carcinoma: systematic review and economic analysis. Health Technol Assess 2007;11(34):1–206.

69. Lok AS, Sterling RK, Everhart JE, et al. Des-gamma-carboxy prothrombin and alpha-fetoprotein as biomarkers for the early detection of hepatocellular carcinoma. Gastroenterology 2010;138(2):493–502.

70. Figueras J, Ibanez L, Ramos E, et al. Selection criteria for liver transplantation in early-stage hepatocellular carcinoma with cirrhosis: results of a multicenter study. Liver Transpl 2001;7(10):877–83.

71. Yao FY, Ferrell L, Bass NM, et al. Liver transplantation for hepatocellular carcinoma: expansion of the tumor size limits does not adversely impact survival. Hepatology 2001;33(6):1394–403.

72. Xu R, Hajdu CH. Wilson disease and hepatocellular carcinoma. Gastroenterol Hepatol (N Y) 2008;4(6):438–9.

73. Davenport MS, Khalatbari S, Dillman JR, et al. Contrast material-induced nephrotoxicity and intravenous low-osmolality iodinated contrast material. Radiology 2013;267(1):94–105.

74. Jha RC, Mitchell DG, Weinreb JC, et al. LI-RADS categorization of benign and likely benign findings in patients at risk of hepatocellular carcinoma: a pictorial atlas. AJR Am J Roentgenol 2014;203(1):W48–69.

75. Mitchell DG, Bruix J, Sherman M, et al. LI-RADS (Liver Imaging Reporting and Data System): summary, discussion, and consensus of the LI-RADS Management Working Group and future directions. Hepatology 2015;61(3):1056–65.

76. Mazzaferro V, Regalia E, Doci R, et al. Liver transplantation for the treatment of small hepatocellular carcinomas in patients with cirrhosis. N Engl J Med 1996; 334(11):693–9.

77. Okuda K, Ohtsuki T, Obata H, et al. Natural history of hepatocellular carcinoma and prognosis in relation to treatment. Study of 850 patients. Cancer 1985;56(4): 918–28.

78. A new prognostic system for hepatocellular carcinoma: a retrospective study of 435 patients: the Cancer of the Liver Italian Program (CLIP) investigators. Hepatology 1998;28(3):751–5.

79. Chevret S, Trinchet JC, Mathieu D, et al. A new prognostic classification for predicting survival in patients with hepatocellular carcinoma. Groupe d'Etude et de Traitement du Carcinome Hepatocellulaire. J Hepatol 1999;31(1):133–41.

80. Forner A, Llovet JM, Bruix J. Hepatocellular carcinoma. Lancet 2012;379(9822): 1245–55.

81. Leung TW, Tang AM, Zee B, et al. Construction of the Chinese University Prognostic Index for hepatocellular carcinoma and comparison with the TNM staging system, the Okuda staging system, and the Cancer of the Liver Italian Program staging system: a study based on 926 patients. Cancer 2002;94(6):1760–9.

82. Ikai I, Takayasu K, Omata M, et al. A modified Japan integrated stage score for prognostic assessment in patients with hepatocellular carcinoma. J Gastroenterol 2006;41(9):884–92.

83. Chapman WC, Klintmalm G, Hemming A, et al. Surgical treatment of hepatocellular carcinoma in North America: can hepatic resection still be justified? J Am Coll Surg 2015;220(4):628–37.

84. Hemming AW, Scudamore CH, Shackleton CR, et al. Indocyanine green clearance as a predictor of successful hepatic resection in cirrhotic patients. Am J Surg 1992;163(5):515–8.

85. Bruix J, Castells A, Bosch J, et al. Surgical resection of hepatocellular carcinoma in cirrhotic patients: prognostic value of preoperative portal pressure. Gastroenterology 1996;111(4):1018–22.

86. Llovet JM, Schwartz M, Mazzaferro V. Resection and liver transplantation for hepatocellular carcinoma. Semin Liver Dis 2005;25(2):181–200.

87. Bismuth H, Majno PE, Adam R. Liver transplantation for hepatocellular carcinoma. Semin Liver Dis 1999;19(3):311–22.

88. Llovet JM, Fuster J, Bruix J. Intention-to-treat analysis of surgical treatment for early hepatocellular carcinoma: resection versus transplantation. Hepatology 1999;30(6):1434–40.

89. Hemming AW, Cattral MS, Reed AI, et al. Liver transplantation for hepatocellular carcinoma. Ann Surg 2001;233(5):652–9.

90. Mazzaferro V, Llovet JM, Miceli R, et al. Predicting survival after liver transplantation in patients with hepatocellular carcinoma beyond the Milan criteria: a retrospective, exploratory analysis. Lancet Oncol 2009;10(1):35–43.
91. Jonas S, Bechstein WO, Steinmuller T, et al. Vascular invasion and histopathologic grading determine outcome after liver transplantation for hepatocellular carcinoma in cirrhosis. Hepatology 2001;33(5):1080–6.
92. Chapman WC, Majella Doyle MB, Stuart JE, et al. Outcomes of neoadjuvant transarterial chemoembolization to downstage hepatocellular carcinoma before liver transplantation. Ann Surg 2008;248(4):617–25.
93. Herrero JI, Sangro B, Pardo F, et al. Liver transplantation in patients with hepatocellular carcinoma across Milan criteria. Liver Transpl 2008;14(3):272–8.
94. Raj A, McCall J, Gane E. Validation of the "Metroticket" predictor in a cohort of patients transplanted for predominantly HBV-related hepatocellular carcinoma. J Hepatol 2011;55(5):1063–8.
95. Lei JY, Wang WT, Yan LN. "Metroticket" predictor for assessing liver transplantation to treat hepatocellular carcinoma: a single-center analysis in mainland China. World J Gastroenterol 2013;19(44):8093–8.
96. Clavien PA, Lesurtel M, Bossuyt PM, et al. Recommendations for liver transplantation for hepatocellular carcinoma: an international consensus conference report. Lancet Oncol 2012;13(1):e11–22.
97. Gordon-Weeks AN, Snaith A, Petrinic T, et al. Systematic review of outcome of downstaging hepatocellular cancer before liver transplantation in patients outside the Milan criteria. Br J Surg 2011;98(9):1201–8.
98. Toso C, Mentha G, Kneteman NM, et al. The place of downstaging for hepatocellular carcinoma. J Hepatol 2010;52(6):930–6.
99. Shiina S. Image-guided percutaneous ablation therapies for hepatocellular carcinoma. J Gastroenterol 2009;44(Suppl 19):122–31.
100. Bouza C, Lopez-Cuadrado T, Alcazar R, et al. Meta-analysis of percutaneous radiofrequency ablation versus ethanol injection in hepatocellular carcinoma. BMC Gastroenterol 2009;9:31.
101. Thomson KR, Cheung W, Ellis SJ, et al. Investigation of the safety of irreversible electroporation in humans. J Vasc Interv Radiol 2011;22(5):611–21.
102. Llovet JM, Bruix J. Systematic review of randomized trials for unresectable hepatocellular carcinoma: chemoembolization improves survival. Hepatology 2003;37(2):429–42.
103. Takayasu K, Arii S, Kudo M, et al. Superselective transarterial chemoembolization for hepatocellular carcinoma. Validation of treatment algorithm proposed by Japanese guidelines. J Hepatol 2012;56(4):886–92.
104. Terzi E, Golfieri R, Piscaglia F, et al. Response rate and clinical outcome of HCC after first and repeated cTACE performed "on demand". J Hepatol 2012;57(6):1258–67.
105. Matsui O, Miyayama S, Sanada J, et al. Interventional oncology: new options for interstitial treatments and intravascular approaches: superselective TACE using iodized oil for HCC: rationale, technique and outcome. J Hepatobiliary Pancreat Sci 2010;17(4):407–9.
106. Lammer J, Malagari K, Vogl T, et al. Prospective randomized study of doxorubicin-eluting-bead embolization in the treatment of hepatocellular carcinoma: results of the PRECISION V study. Cardiovasc Intervent Radiol 2010;33(1):41–52.
107. Italian Association for the Study of the Liver (AISF), AISF Expert Panel, AISF Coordinating Committee, et al. Position paper of the Italian Association for the

Study of the Liver (AISF): the multidisciplinary clinical approach to hepatocellular carcinoma. Dig Liver Dis 2013;45(9):712–23.

108. Llovet JM, Ricci S, Mazzaferro V, et al. Sorafenib in advanced hepatocellular carcinoma. N Engl J Med 2008;359(4):378–90.

109. Cheng AL, Kang YK, Chen Z, et al. Efficacy and safety of sorafenib in patients in the Asia-Pacific region with advanced hepatocellular carcinoma: a phase III randomised, double-blind, placebo-controlled trial. Lancet Oncol 2009;10(1): 25–34.

110. Lencioni R, Llovet JM, Han G, et al. Sorafenib or placebo plus TACE with doxorubicin-eluting beads for intermediate stage HCC: the SPACE trial. J Hepatol 2016;64(5):1090–8.

111. Bruix J, Takayama T, Mazzaferro V, et al. Adjuvant sorafenib for hepatocellular carcinoma after resection or ablation (STORM): a phase 3, randomised, double-blind, placebo-controlled trial. Lancet Oncol 2015;16(13):1344–54.

The Management of Hepatitis B in Liver Transplant Recipients

Sammy Saab, MD, MPH[a,b,]*, Ping-yu Chen, MD[b], Clara E. Saab, BA[a],
Myron J. Tong, MD, PhD[a,c]

KEYWORDS

- Hepatitis B • Cirrhosis • Liver transplant • Antiviral therapy

KEY POINTS

- Hepatitis B is an important indication for liver transplant.
- Clinical outcomes for patients transplanted for hepatitis B have significantly improved.
- The approach to managing hepatitis B in liver transplant recipients begins before surgery.
- Emerging data suggest a diminishing role of hepatitis B immunoglobulin in favor of newer-generation all-oral antiviral therapy.

INTRODUCTION

Chronic hepatitis B (CHB) is a worldwide health concern. It has been estimated that it affects up to 240 million people in the world, with the highest prevalence found in Asia and Africa.[1] Patients infected with CHB are at risk for liver-related complications such as cirrhosis, decompensated liver disease, and hepatocellular carcinoma (HCC).[2–4] In select patients with HCC and/or decompensated liver disease, orthotopic liver transplant (OLT) is considered the definitive treatment. However, in the absence of antiviral prophylaxis or treatment, hepatitis B virus (HBV) reinfection may occur in 75% to 80% of patients who undergo liver transplant (LT), which significantly affects their survival.[5] The mortality is 50% 2 years after LT without antiviral prophylaxis.[6] One of the leading theories explaining the propensity for the high rate of HBV reinfection after LT is the direct stimulation on the glucocorticoid responsive enhancer region of the HBV genome resulting in enhanced viral replication by

Disclosure: The authors have nothing to disclose.
[a] Department of Surgery, University of California at Los Angeles, Los Angeles, CA, USA; [b] Department of Medicine, University of California at Los Angeles, Los Angeles, CA, USA; [c] Huntington Medical Research Institutes, Pasadena, CA, USA
* Corresponding author. Pfleger Liver Institute, UCLA Medical Center, 200 Medical Plaza, Suite 214, Los Angeles, CA 90095.
E-mail address: SSaab@mednet.ucla.edu

corticosteroids.[7,8] Thus, the primary goal in the management of patients transplanted for HBV is to prevent reinfection.

There are several risk factors for HBV reinfection following LT (**Box 1**). One of the most important risk factors for reinfection is the hepatitis B viral level at the time of transplant, with a value greater than 20,000 IU/mL associated with an increased risk for reinfection.[9,10] Other risk factors for reinfection include the presence of antiviral drug resistance before transplant and noncompliance with antiviral therapy.[11] Several studies have also reported that HCC recurrence in LT recipients was independently associated with increased risk of HBV recurrence.[12,13] The detection of covalently closed circular DNA in HCC cells suggests the possibility of viral replication in liver tumor cells, which acts as a viral reservoir and may in part explain the association between HCC and HBV recurrence.[14] However, patients transplanted for fulminant HBV seem to be at a low risk of HBV reinfection.[15,16]

Although HBV-related liver disease was previously a relative and sometimes absolute contraindication for LT, the past decade has seen significant improvement in the outcomes for patients with HBV. Not only has the need for transplant decreased but patient survival after LT is higher than most other indications for transplant.[17–19] At present, HBV accounts for 5% to 10% of LTs in the United States and Europe,[19,20] but is the leading cause for LT in Asia.[21,22] This article discusses the current guidelines and therapies for pretransplant and posttransplant management of patients with CHB.

ANTIVIRAL THERAPY

There are several nucleoside/nucleotide analogues (NAs) approved for treating CHB, of which 3 are nucleoside analogues (lamivudine [LAM], telbivudine, and entecavir [ETV]) and 2 are nucleotide analogues.[23,24] Nucleotide analogues differ from nucleoside analogues by the addition of 3 phosphate groups. Both analogues target the reverse transcription of HBV and achieve inhibition of HBV replication via incorporation into viral HBV DNA causing DNA chain termination.[23] The NAs differ in the viral suppression potency and genetic barrier resistance. The early-generation NAs (LAM, adefovir [ADV], and telbivudine) had lower rates of viral suppression and/or higher risk of resistance. In contrast, the newer NAs (ETV and tenofovir [TDV]) are potent antiviral agents and both have a high genetic barrier to drug resistance.[25] ETV and tenofovir are currently first-line therapies for CHB.[23,26] The oral doses of all NAs need to be adjusted according to the level of creatinine clearance because of the risk of lactic acidosis in patients with compromised kidney function.[27] Pegylated interferon should be avoided in LT recipients with cirrhosis because of the risk of decompensation and graft loss.

Box 1
Risk factors for recurrent hepatitis B in LT recipients

High hepatitis B viral levels before LT

Increased hepatitis B surface antigen levels.

Coinfection with human immunodeficiency virus or hepatitis C

Noncompliance

Presence of antiviral drug resistance

Presence of hepatocellular carcinoma before LT

Hepatitis B E antigen positive

No posttransplant hepatitis B prophylaxis

TREATMENT OF HEPATITIS B INFECTION BEFORE LIVER TRANSPLANT

Several studies have examined the role of NAs in the treatment of both compensated and decompensated liver disease. The results of recent systematic reviews and meta-analyses have highlighted not only the possibility of cirrhosis regression in patients with compensated cirrhosis but also the improvement in liver function in patients with decompensated liver disease[28–34] For instance, the use of both ETV and tenofovir has been associated with cirrhosis regression in patients with HBV.[35–37] The resolution of fibrosis seems to be related to duration of viral suppression, with greater fibrosis improvement occurring over longer periods of follow-up.[34] Equally important, the use of NAs was associated with improvement of liver function estimated by either Child-Turcotte-Pugh (CTP) or Model for End-stage Liver Disease (MELD) score.[38,39] For instance, Liaw and colleagues[38] studied 191 patients with CTP scores of at least 7 for 96 weeks who were randomized to receive either ETV or ADV therapy.[38] A reduction of at least 2 points in the CTP score was shown in 35% of patients taking ETV versus 27% of patients receiving ADV. The mean reductions from baseline MELD scores in ETV-treated and ADV-treated patients were 2.6 and 1.7 respectively at week 48. Another trial reported 112 patients with HBV and decompensated cirrhosis who were treated with ETV, TDV, or tenofovir-emtricitabine. The investigators noted a decrease in CTP score of at least 2 points as well as a median decrease of 2 MELD score points in all treatment groups.[40]

TREATMENT OF HEPATITIS B INFECTION AFTER LIVER TRANSPLANT

The management of HBV in LT recipients should be initiated before surgery, because high levels of pretransplant HBV load predicted posttransplant recurrence.[41] LT candidates should be on an NA and ideally have undetectable or near-undetectable HBV viral levels at the time of LT.[42,43] After transplant, there are several strategies to prevent reinfection (**Fig. 1**). One of the most popular posttransplant strategies is the

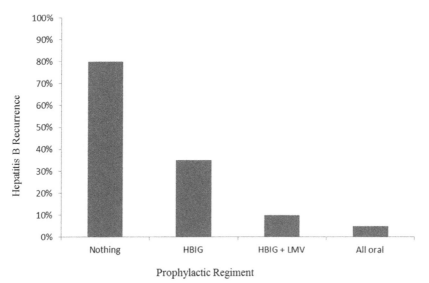

Fig. 1. Evolution of hepatitis B prophylaxis in liver transplant recipients. HBIG, hepatitis B immunoglobulin; LAM, lamivudine.

combination of hepatitis B immunoglobulin (HBIG) and an NA. However, there is no generalized consensus on the proper use of HBIG.[15] There is increasing interest in using oral therapy for several reasons, including convenience, efficacy, and tolerability (**Table 1**).

Hepatitis B Immunoglobulin Monotherapy

HBIG is a polyclonal antibody to Hepatitis B Surface Antigen (HBsAg) derived from pooled human plasma.[44] Previous studies suggested that antibodies to HBsAg bind to and neutralize circulating virions, which in turn prevent graft reinfection.[45] Although its mechanism of action is not completely understood, the HBIG-virion complex may prevent hepatocyte infection. The efficacy of HBIG in prevention of recurrent HBV infection after OLT was first shown by 2 important reports by Samuel and colleagues.[16,46] In a 1993 study, patients who received more than 6 months of high-dose HBIG monotherapy had a 33% risk of recurrence compared with a 75% risk of recurrence in patients who received none or less than 6 months of HBIG therapy.[16] In addition, prevention of HBV recurrence in OLT recipients with HBIG significantly reduced morbidity and mortality after LT.[47]

Although HBIG was initially developed to be administered parentally, this mode is costly and inconvenient. Moreover, long-term use of HBIG monotherapy may also result in development of genetic HBV mutants; the most common mutation reported is the substitution of glycine by arginine at codon 145 of the HBV surface protein.[48]

Multiple strategies have been developed to reduce the dose of HBIG. One dosing method is an individualized tailored approach that titrates HBIG dose according to the patient's anti-HBs titer. Most institutions define an antibodies to hepatitis B surface antigen (anti-HBs) titer greater than 100 IU/L as protective.[15] Other studies have also shown that antiviral therapy with nucleoside/nucleotide analogues before OLT decreases the risk of HBV reinfection by reducing the amount of circulating virus at the time of LT.[49] An alternative mode of administrating HBIG has been through the intramuscular (IM) route. IM administration of HBIG has also been shown to be as effective as the intravenous (IV) route in producing anti-HBs titers in LT recipients.[47] Thus, not only is IM HBIG as effective as IV HBIG but IM HBIG is more convenient and less costly. There is approximately a 60% cost reduction when using the IM rather than the IV

Table 1		
Comparison of hepatitis B immunoglobulin nucleosides/nucleotides		
	HBIG	**Nucleosides/Nucleotides**
Administration	IV/IM	Oral
Setting	Office	Home
Standardization	No	Yes
Frequency	Monthly	Every day
Adverse effects	Injection site	None Lactic acidosis?
Resistance	Viral breakthrough as monotherapy	Yes, with first generation
Mechanism	Neutralize antigen?	Inhibit viral replication
Monitoring	Anti-HB titers	Renal function
Costs	↑↑↑	↑↑

Abbreviations: HB, hepatitis B; HBIG, hepatitis B immunoglobulin; IV, intravenous; IM, intramuscular.

route.[50] Another mode of administration that is currently under study but not yet available is the subcutaneous (SC) route. In a study by Singham and colleagues,[51] the mode of administration of HBIG was changed from IM to SC in 12 LT recipients. All recipients were able to maintain titers of anti-HBs at greater than 100 IU/mL and there were no cases of HBV reinfection. Similar results were noted by Yahyazadeh and colleagues[52] in their study of 23 LT recipients. The main advantage to SC HBIG is the potential for self-administration at home, decreased cost, and decreased adverse side effects. However, only the IV and IM versions of HBIG are currently available.

However, HBIG alone as prophylaxis is no longer used because of the high risk of HBV recurrence.[15]

Combination of Hepatitis B Immunoglobulin and Antiviral Agents

The combination of HBIG with an NA is considered by many physicians to be the mainstay of prophylactic regimens to prevent HBV recurrence in LT recipients. The most studied combination is LAM and HBIG. The results of a meta-analysis of 2 prospective and 4 retrospective studies suggested that this combination therapy was associated with significantly reduced HBV-related and all-cause mortality after transplant.[53] Two systematic reviews and meta-analyses by Katz and colleagues[54,55] in 2010 also showed that HBIG in combination with LAM was superior to either HBIG or LAM monotherapy. Because of their different mechanisms of action, HBIG and antivirals work in a synergistic manner to prevent HBV recurrence.

The main concern with the use of LAM is the high likelihood of developing drug resistance.[56] Thus, in patients with LAM resistance, other nucleoside analogues used as monotherapy should be avoided because of cross-resistance. The substitution of ADV for LAM in combination therapy with HBIG showed acceptable outcomes in transplant recipients with LAM-resistant variants. The use of HBIG with ADV in LAM-resistant patients with mutations in the tyrosine-methionine-aspartate-aspartate (YMDD) resulted in a reduced recurrence rate of 6% to 9% at 2 years after transplant.[57] A systematic review by Cholongitas and colleagues[58] compared high-dose HBIG (10,000 IU/d) versus low-dose HBIG (<10,000IU/d) in combination with either LAM or ADV. The investigators concluded that recurrence was lower in patients on high-dose HBIG therapy with LAM but that dose variation in patients treated with the ADV and HBIG combination had no impact on recurrent HBV infection.

As in the general population, the use of ETV and tenofovir disoproxil fumarate (TDF) has become first-line oral therapies for HBV in LT recipients because of their high genetic barrier to resistance and strong potency to suppress viral replication.[59] In a systemic review by Cholongitas and colleagues[58] of 17 studies on LT recipients with HBV, recipients treated with combination therapy with HBIG and either ETV or TDF were significantly less likely to develop HBV recurrence than recipients treated with combination therapy with HBIG and LAM. Viral suppression was also maintained when recipients were treated with ETV and varying the doses of HBIG.[60] The use of ETV was effective in maintaining viral suppression, even in recipients who experienced a reappearance of HBsAg.

Because of the inconvenience and cost of continual HBIG administration and emerging data suggesting that recipients' outcomes remain good even after reemergence of HBsAg as long as viral suppression is achieved, there is growing interest in discontinuing HBIG.

Withdrawal of Hepatitis B Immunoglobulin After Combination Therapy

There are several studies assessing the impact of using oral combination therapy without HBIG in patients who received an LT for HBV[61–78] (Table 2). Most studies

Table 2
Newer nucleosides/nucleotides after hepatitis B immune globulin withdrawal, for prevention of hepatitis B virus recurrence after LT

Author (Reference)	Number	Study Design	Study Population	Antiviral Regiment	Mean Follow-up	Outcome	Definition of Recurrence
Cholongitas et al,[61] 2012	47	PC	4.5% HBV DNA+	HBIG for ≥12 mo then 23 LAM + ADV, 5 LAM + TDF, 10 TDF only, and 9 ETV only	24 mo	0% recurrence 6.3% HBsAg+ 100% HBV DNA−	Evidence of clinical recurrence
Nath et al,[62] 2006	14	PC	100% HBsAg+ 79% HBV DNA+	LAM + HBIG × 7 d after LT then ADV + LAM only	14.1 mo	0% recurrence 7% HBsAg+ At least 1 with detectable HBV DNA level	—
Wong et al,[63] 2007	2	PC	50% HBV DNA− 50% unknown	1 LAM to LAM + ADV and 1 LAM to FTC + TDF when LAM resistance was detected HBIG discontinued 12–26 mo	45–50 mo	50% recurrence 50% HBsAg+ 100% HBV DNA−	Positive HBsAg or HBV DNA greater than or equal to 5 log copies/mL on 2 consecutive occasions
Angus et al,[64] 2008	16	Randomized Open label	28% HBV DNA+	>12 mo of HBIG + LAM before ADV + LAM only	24 mo	0% recurrence 6% HBsAg+ 100% HBV DNA−	Positive HBV DNA
Gane et al,[65] 2013	20	PC	Median HBV DNA 4log10 IU/mL	HBIG × 7 d after LT then LAM + ADV only	57 mo	0% recurrence 0% HBsAg+ 100% HBV DNA−	Positive HBV DNA and HBsAg
Teperman et al,[67] 2013	18	Randomized phase 2	100% HBV DNA−	24 wk FTC + TDF + HBIG then FTC + TDF only	72 wk	0% recurrence 0% HBsAg+ 100% HBV DNA−	Positive HBV DNA and HBsAg
Stravitz et al,[68] 2012	21	PC	100% HBV DNA−	HBIG + NA ≥6 mo then TDF + FTC only	31.1 mo	0% recurrence 14% HBsAg+ 100% HBV DNA−	Positive HBV DNA

Study	No.	Type	Patient characteristics	Treatment	Follow-up	Outcome	Definition of recurrence
Tanaka et al,[69] 2014	24	PC	50% HBV DNA <2.1 log copies/mL	15 TDF only and 9 LAM + TDF HBIG discontinued after 12 mo	29.1 mo	0% recurrence 0% HBsAg+ 100% HBV DNA−	Positive HBsAg and HBV DNA
Wesdorp et al,[70] 2013	17	PC	94% HBV DNA−	HBIG ± NA ≥6 mo then TDF + FTC only	2 y	0% recurrence 6% HBsAg+ 100% HBV DNA−	Positive HBV DNA and HBsAg
Khemichian et al,[71] 2015	26	PC	unknown	HBIG with 1 NA then if HBsAg− after 1 y, changed to 2 NA monotherapy without HBIG	31.9 mo	8% recurrence 8% HBsAg+ 100% HBV DNA−	Positive HBsAg
Fernandez et al,[72] 2015	58	PC	15 HBV DNA+	HBIG + NA for ≥12 mo then 31 TDF and 27 ETV only	28 mo	0% recurrence 8.6% HBsAg+ 100% HBV DNA−	Evidence of clinical recurrence
Saab et al,[73] 2011	61	RC	42 with available pre-LT DNA (9 of 42 with HBV DNA+)	HBIG + 1nucleoside (LAM/ETV) ≥12 mo then 2 nucleoside + 1 nucleotide (TDF/ADV) only	15 mo	3.3% recurrence 3.3% HBsAg+ 100% HBV DNA−	Positive HBsAg
Neff et al,[74] 2007	10	RC	100% HBV DNA−	HBIG + LAM ≥6 mo then LAM + ADV	31 mo	0% recurrence 0% HBsAg+ 100% HBV DNA−	Positive HBV DNA, HBsAg, and abnormal liver tests
Weber et al,[75] 2010	12	RC	100% HBsAg+ 5 of 12 unknown HBV DNA, 1 of 12 HBV DNA+	HBIG + NA for median 62.8 mo after LT + HBV vaccine then 7 LAM, 2 ADV, 3 ETV only	27.4 mo	0% recurrence	HBV DNA >10(4) copies/mL on 2 consecutive occasions or viral recurrence with increased transaminase levels

(continued on next page)

Table 2
(continued)

Author (Reference)	Number	Study Design	Study Population	Antiviral Regiment	Mean Follow-up	Outcome	Definition of Recurrence
McGonigal et al,[76] 2013	4	Case series	25% HBV DNA >300IU/mL	HBIG + NA then TDF/FTC only	Up to 15 mo	0% recurrence 0% HBsAg+ 100% HBV DNA–	Positive HBV DNA
Singer et al,[77] 2015	13	PC	100% HBsAg+	HBIG × 2 doses at LT then TDF or ETV only	23 mo	7.7% recurrence	Positive HBV DNA of 16 IU/mL with HCC
Akcam et al,[78] 2015	12	PC	Unknown	HBIG then 6 TDF and 6 ETV only	16–27 mo	0% recurrence 0% HBsAg+ 100% HBV DNA–	—

Abbreviations: FTC, emtricitabine; HBIG, human B immunoglobulin; NA, nucleoside/nucleotide analogue; PC, prospective cohort; RC, retrospective cohort.

define recurrent HBV as detection of HBV DNA. All studies used a combination of a nucleoside and nucleotide analogue, but the minimal duration of HBIG before its withdrawal has varied. One of the earliest published studies was by Nath and colleagues.[62] The investigators noted continual viral suppression using the combination of ADV and LAM in 14 recipients after 7 days of HBIG. One patient remained HBsAg positive but had negative HBV DNA at a mean of 14.1 months' follow-up.[62] Another study by Wong and colleagues[63] showed the possibility of HBIG withdrawal. The investigators discontinued HBIG at a median of 26 months after LT and noted no evidence of HBV recurrence except in 1 of 25 recipients, who was not compliant with the NA regimen. Angus and colleagues[64] showed no negative impact on patient survival when ADV was substituted for HBIG in recipients who had previously been treated for least 12 months with HBIG and LAM. Also, the combination of LAM and ADV was effective in preventing recurrent infection when antiviral therapy was initiated before transplant and HBIG was used for a limited period of time after transplant.[65] Moreover, the investigators suggested that HBIG may not be necessary in recipients treated with the combination of LAM and ADV provided that their viral load was less than 3log10 IU/mL before OLT.

Oral Therapy Without Hepatitis B Immunoglobulin

There is very limited experience but increasing interest in using oral antiviral therapy alone without HBIG prophylaxis after LT[60,65,79–82] (**Table 3**). Although the outcomes seem promising, interpretation of the results and the adverse effect profiles are confounded by small single-center cohort designs, mixed NA regimens, and short follow-up periods. For instance, Genzini and colleagues[79] described 21 patients treated with LAM, LAM + ADV, or ETV before transplant. Patient survival was 90%, with 1 patient lost to follow-up and 1 graft loss because of HBV recurrence from medical noncompliance. During a mean follow-up of 19.5 months, HBV viral suppression was shown in 15 LT recipients. In a larger study of 75 LT recipients using different NA treatments (ETV, n = 42; LAM + ADV, n = 19; TDF, n = 12; and ETV + TDF, n = 2) without HBIG, Wadhawan and colleagues[80] showed HBV recurrence in 8% of recipients (6 of 75), 5 of which were caused by lack of adherence to the treatment regimen.

VACCINATION AGAINST HEPATITIS B

There have been some studies investigating the use of active immunization with recombinant hepatitis B vaccines in an attempt to reduce the need for long-term HBIG. Successful HBV vaccine induction was first reported by Sánchez-Fueyo and colleagues[83]; 82% of patients responded to the vaccine after LT. However, subsequent studies could not reproduce the same results.[84–87] At this time, the studies have contradictory results and hepatitis B vaccination is not currently recommended for use as prophylaxis for post-LT patients.

HEPATITIS B CORE POSITIVE GRAFTS

The number of patients waiting for LT remains higher than the number of transplants performed.[88,89] Thus, there has been a demand to use expanded criteria organs for transplant.[88] One type of expanded criteria organ graft is a graft exposed to hepatitis B (anti–HB core [HBc] positive) but without evidence of immunity (anti-HBc negative). Early experience with anti-HBc–positive grafts was unsuccessful in recipients without HBV immunity (anti-HBs negative) because of HBV reactivation, which affected patient survival.[90] However, the use of anti-HBc–positive grafts does not affect the outcomes of recipients who have HBV immunity or of recipients receiving prophylaxis.[91–93]

Table 3
Nucleosides/nucleotides without HBIG for prevention of hepatitis B virus recurrence after LT

Author (Reference)	Number	Study Design	Study Population	Antiviral Regiment	Mean Follow-up	Outcome	Definition of Recurrence
Perrillo et al,[60] 2013	1	RC	100% HBV DNA−	ETV only	2 y	0% recurrence 6% HBsAg+	HBV DNA ≥300 copies/mL
Gane et al,[65] 2013	18	PC	100% HBV DNA−	LAM + ADV only	22 mo	0% recurrence 0% HBsAg+ 100% HBV DNA−	Positive HBV DNA
Genzini et al,[79] 2010	19	PC	28.5% HBV DNA−	11 LAM, 3 LAM + ADV, and 5 ETV only	19.5 mo	1 graft loss caused by poor access	—
Wadhawan et al,[80] 2013	75	PC	100% HBV DNA<2000 IU/mL	19 LAM + ADV, 2 ETV + TDF, 12 TDF, 42 ETV only	21 mo	8% recurrence 8% HBsAg+	Positive HBV DNA 6 mo after LT
Fung et al,[81] 2011	80	PC	26% HBV DNA−	ETV only	26 mo	22.5% recurrence 22.5% HBsAg+ 94% HBV−	Positive HBsAg
Ahn et al,[82] 2011	1	RC	Not available	TDF	Not available	0% recurrence 0% HBsAg+ 100% HBV DNA−	Positive HBsAg and HBV DNA

Reactivation can be prevented in recipients without immunity if HBV prophylaxis is used. In a systemic review by Saab and colleagues,[94] the incidence of de novo hepatitis B infection was 2.7% in patients receiving LAM-only prophylaxis versus 3.6% in patients receiving HBIG and LAM combination therapy. The doses and duration of HBIG in the combination therapies was highly variable. It was concluded that published studies have not shown that combination therapy was more effective than LAM monotherapy.[94] However, given the risk of drug resistance with LAM, there is increasing interest in using TDV or ETV for HBV prophylaxis in recipients transplanted with anti-HBc–positive grafts.

TREATMENT OF HEPATITIS B INFECTION IN LIVER TRANSPLANT RECIPIENTS

LT recipients are at risk of HBV infection through high-risk contact, anti-HBc–positive donor organs without adequate prophylaxis, and breakthrough despite posttransplant prophylaxis. Hepatitis B infection is defined as the detection of circulating levels of HBsAg with or without measureable HBV DNA viral titers or histologic evidence of liver disease. The treatments for HBV in LT recipients is the same as is recommended for immunocompetent individuals.[95] The choice of which NA depends on which regimen the transplant recipients had previously received. In LT recipients who failed a combination of HBIG and NA, the HBIG is generally discontinued and a second NA of a different class (nucleotide or nucleoside) is used according to American Association for the Study of Liver Diseases guidelines.

SUMMARY

LT is now a fairly safe and established indication for patients with CHB, mainly because of the development and use of HBIG and oral antivirals for prophylaxis. The combination of low-dose HBIG and antivirals is currently considered the standard prophylaxis regimen to prevent post-LT recurrence of hepatitis B. The important remaining issues are related to the long-term cost of HBIG and the risk of escape HBV mutants. Strategies for prevention of HBV after LT are constantly evolving and improving. With the availability of new NAs, new post-LT strategies also should emerge.

REFERENCES

1. Ott JJ, Stevens GA, Groeger J, et al. Global epidemiology of hepatitis B virus infection: new estimates of age-specific HBsAg seroprevalence and endemicity. Vaccine 2012;30(12):2212–9.
2. Iloeje UH, Yang HI, Chen CJ. Natural history of chronic hepatitis B: what exactly has REVEAL revealed? Liver Int 2012;32(9):1333–41.
3. Fattovich G, Bortolotti F, Donato F. Natural history of chronic hepatitis B: special emphasis on disease progression and prognostic factors. J Hepatol 2008; 48(2):335–52.
4. Yim HJ, Lok AS. Natural history of chronic hepatitis B virus infection: what we knew in 1981 and what we know in 2005. Hepatology 2006;43(2 Suppl 1): S173–81.
5. O'Grady JG, Smith HM, Davies SE, et al. Hepatitis B virus reinfection after orthotopic liver transplantation. Serological and clinical implications. J Hepatol 1992; 14(1):104–11.
6. Ishigami M, Ogura Y, Hirooka Y, et al. Change of strategies and future perspectives against hepatitis B virus recurrence after liver transplantation. World J Gastroenterol 2015;21(36):10290–8.

7. Tur-Kaspa R, Shaul Y, Moore DD, et al. The glucocorticoid receptor recognizes a specific nucleotide sequence in hepatitis B virus DNA causing increased activity of the HBV enhancer. Virology 1988;167(2):630–3.

8. McMillan JS, Shaw T, Angus PW, et al. Effect of immunosuppressive and antiviral agents on hepatitis B virus replication in vitro. Hepatology 1995;22(1):36–43.

9. Tung BY, Kowdley KV. Hepatitis B and liver transplantation. Clin Infect Dis 2015; 41:1461–6.

10. Roche B, Roque-Afonso AM, Nevens F, et al. Rational basis for optimizing short and long-term hepatitis B virus prophylaxis post liver transplantation: role of hepatitis B immune globulin. Transplantation 2015;99(7):1321–34.

11. Xie SB, Zhu JY, Ying Z, et al. Prevention and risk factors of the HBV recurrence after orthotopic liver transplantation: 160 cases follow-up study. Transplantation 2010;90(7):786–90.

12. Faria LC, Gigou M, Roque-Afonso AM, et al. Hepatocellular carcinoma is associated with an increased risk of hepatitis B virus recurrence after liver transplantation. Gastroenterology 2008;134(7):1890–9.

13. Saab S, Yeganeh M, Nguyen K, et al. Recurrence of hepatocellular carcinoma and hepatitis B reinfection in hepatitis B surface antigen-positive patients after liver transplantation. Liver Transpl 2009;15(11):1525–34.

14. Kumar R, Pérez-Del-Pulgar S, Testoni B, et al. Clinical relevance of the study of hepatitis B virus covalently closed circular DNA. Liver Int 2016;36(Suppl 1):72–7.

15. Degertekin B, Han SH, Keeffe EB, et al, NIH HBV-OLT Study Group. Impact of virologic breakthrough and HBIG regimen on hepatitis B recurrence after liver transplantation. Am J Transplant 2010;10(8):1823–33.

16. Samuel D, Muller R, Alexander G, et al. Liver transplantation in European patients with the hepatitis B surface antigen. N Engl J Med 1993;329(25):1842–7.

17. Kim WR, Poterucha JJ, Kremers WK, et al. Outcome of liver transplantation for hepatitis B in the United States. Liver Transpl 2004;10(8):968–74.

18. Al-Hamoudi W, Elsiesy H, Bendahmash A, et al. Liver transplantation for hepatitis B virus: decreasing indication and changing trends. World J Gastroenterol 2015; 21(26):8140–7.

19. Kim WR, Terrault NA, Pedersen RA, et al. Trends in waiting list registration for liver transplantation for viral hepatitis in the United States. Gastroenterology 2009; 137(5):1680–6.

20. Burra P, Germani G, Adam R, et al. Liver transplantation for HBV-related cirrhosis in Europe: an ELTR study on evolution and outcomes. J Hepatol 2013;58(2): 287–96.

21. Shukla A, Vadeyar H, Rela M, et al. Liver transplantation: east versus west. J Clin Exp Hepatol 2013;3(3):243–53.

22. Lee SG, Moon DB, Hwang S, et al. Liver transplantation in Korea: past, present, and future. Transplant Proc 2015;47(3):705–8.

23. Jafri SM, Lok AS. Antiviral therapy for chronic hepatitis B. Clin Liver Dis 2010; 14(3):425–38.

24. Lok AS, McMahon BJ, Brown RS Jr, et al. Antiviral therapy for chronic hepatitis B viral infection in adults: a systematic review and meta-analysis. Hepatology 2016; 63(1):284–306.

25. Woo G, Tomlinson G, Nishikawa Y, et al. Tenofovir and entecavir are the most effective antiviral agents for chronic hepatitis B: a systematic review and Bayesian meta-analyses. Gastroenterology 2010;139(4):1218–29.

26. Russo FP, Rodríguez-Castro K, Scribano L, et al. Role of antiviral therapy in the natural history of hepatitis B virus-related chronic liver disease. World J Hepatol 2015;7(8):1097–104.

27. Lok AS, McMahon BJ. Chronic hepatitis B. Hepatology 2007;45(2):507–39.

28. Roche B, Samuel D. Treatment of patients with HBV-related decompensated cirrhosis and liver transplanted patients. Clin Liver Dis 2013;17(3):451–73.

29. Cholongitas E, Papatheodoridis GV, Goulis J, et al. The impact of newer nucleos(t)ide analogues on patients with hepatitis B decompensated cirrhosis. Ann Gastroenterol 2015;28(1):109–17.

30. Jang JW, Choi JY, Kim YS, et al. Long-term effect of antiviral therapy on disease course after decompensation in patients with hepatitis B virus-related cirrhosis. Hepatology 2015;61(6):1809–20.

31. Singal AK, Fontana RJ. Meta-analysis: oral anti-viral agents in adults with decompensated hepatitis B virus cirrhosis. Aliment Pharmacol Ther 2012;35(6):674–89.

32. Honda K, Seike M, Murakami K. Benefits of nucleos(t)ide analog treatments for hepatitis B virus-related cirrhosis. World J Hepatol 2015;7(22):2404–10.

33. Lampertico P, Invernizzi F, Viganò M, et al. The long-term benefits of nucleos(t)ide analogs in compensated HBV cirrhotic patients with no or small esophageal varices: a 12-year prospective cohort study. J Hepatol 2015;63(5):1118–25.

34. Manne V, Akhtar E, Saab S. Cirrhosis regression in patients with viral hepatitis B and C: a systematic review. J Clin Gastroenterol 2014;48:76–8.

35. Calvaruso V, Craxì A. Regression of fibrosis after HBV antiviral therapy. Is cirrhosis reversible? Liver Int 2014;34(Suppl 1):85–90.

36. Chang TT, Liaw YF, Wu SS, et al. Long-term entecavir therapy results in the reversal of fibrosis/cirrhosis and continued histological improvement in patients with chronic hepatitis B. Hepatology 2010;52(3):886–93.

37. Marcellin P, Gane E, Buti M, et al. Regression of cirrhosis during treatment with tenofovir disoproxil fumarate for chronic hepatitis B: a 5-year open-label follow-up study. Lancet 2013;381(9865):468–75.

38. Liaw YF, Raptopoulou-Gigi M, Cheinquer H, et al. Efficacy and safety of entecavir versus adefovir in chronic hepatitis B patients with hepatic decompensation: a randomized, open-label study. Hepatology 2011;54(1):91–100.

39. Shim JH, Lee HC, Kim KM, et al. Efficacy of entecavir in treatment-naïve patients with hepatitis B virus-related decompensated cirrhosis. J Hepatol 2010;52(2):176–82.

40. Liaw YF, Sheen IS, Lee CM, et al. Tenofovir disoproxil fumarate (TDF), emtricitabine/TDF, and entecavir in patients with decompensated chronic hepatitis B liver disease. Hepatology 2011;53(1):62–72.

41. Manne V, Allen RM, Saab S. Strategies for the prevention of recurrent hepatitis B virus infection after liver transplantation. Gastroenterol Hepatol (N Y) 2014;10(3):175–9.

42. Angus PW, Patterson SJ. Liver transplantation for hepatitis B: what is the best hepatitis B immune globulin/antiviral regimen? Liver Transpl 2008;14(Suppl 2):S15–22.

43. Harmancı Ö, Selçuk H, Haberal M. Prophylaxis against recurrence in liver transplantation patients with hepatitis B virus: what is new? J Clin Transl Hepatol 2014;2(4):259–65.

44. Shouval D, Samuel D. Hepatitis B immune globulin to prevent hepatitis B virus graft reinfection following liver transplantation: a concise review. Hepatology 2000;32(6):1189–95.

45. Schilling R, Ijaz S, Davidoff M, et al. Endocytosis of hepatitis B immune globulin into hepatocytes inhibits the secretion of hepatitis B virus surface antigen and virions. J Virol 2003;77(16):8882–92.

46. Samuel D, Bismuth A, Mathieu D, et al. Passive immunoprophylaxis after liver transplantation in HBsAg-positive patients. Lancet 1991;337(8745):813–5.

47. Kasraianfard A, Watt KD, Lindberg L, et al. HBIG remains significant in the era of new potent nucleoside analogues for prophylaxis against hepatitis B recurrence after liver transplantation. Int Rev Immunol 2014. [Epub ahead of print].

48. Park GC, Hwang S, Ahn CS, et al. Analysis of S gene mutation of the hepatitis B virus in adult liver transplant recipients showing resistance to hepatitis B immunoglobulin therapy. Transplant Proc 2013;45(8):3047–51.

49. Dickson RC, Terrault NA, Ishitani M, et al. Protective antibody levels and dose requirements for IV 5% Nabi Hepatitis B immune globulin combined with lamivudine in liver transplantation for hepatitis B-induced end stage liver disease. Liver Transpl 2006;12(1):124–33.

50. Hulstaert E, Verhelst X, Geerts A, et al. Intramuscular hepatitis B immunoglobulins for reinfection control after liver transplantation: a cost-saving alternative. J Comp Eff Res 2015;8:1–7.

51. Singham J, Greanya ED, Lau K, et al. Efficacy of maintenance subcutaneous hepatitis B immune globulin (HBIG) post-transplant for prophylaxis against hepatitis B recurrence. Ann Hepatol 2010;9(2):166–71.

52. Yahyazadeh A, Beckebaum S, Cicinnati V, et al. Efficacy and safety of subcutaneous human HBV-immunoglobulin (Zutectra) in liver transplantation: an open, prospective, single-arm phase III study. Transpl Int 2011;24(5):441–50.

53. Loomba R, Rowley AK, Wesley R, et al. Hepatitis B immunoglobulin and lamivudine improve hepatitis B-related outcomes after liver transplantation: meta-analysis. Clin Gastroenterol Hepatol 2008;6(6):696–700.

54. Katz LH, Paul M, Guy DG, et al. Prevention of recurrent hepatitis B virus infection after liver transplantation: hepatitis B immunoglobulin, antiviral drugs, or both? Systematic review and meta-analysis. Transpl Infect Dis 2010;12(4):292–308.

55. Katz LH, Tur-Kaspa R, Guy DG, et al. Lamivudine or adefovir dipivoxil alone or combined with immunoglobulin for preventing hepatitis B recurrence after liver transplantation. Cochrane Database Syst Rev 2010;(7):CD006005.

56. Liaw YF. Impact of YMDD mutations during lamivudine therapy in patients with chronic hepatitis B. Antivir Chem Chemother 2001;12(Suppl 1):67–71.

57. Perrillo R, Hann HW, Mutimer D, et al. Adefovir dipivoxil added to ongoing lamivudine in chronic hepatitis B with YMDD mutant hepatitis B virus. Gastroenterology 2004;126(1):81–90.

58. Cholongitas E, Goulis J, Akriviadis E, et al. Hepatitis B immunoglobulin and/or nucleos(t)ide analogues for prophylaxis against hepatitis b virus recurrence after liver transplantation: a systematic review. Liver Transpl 2011;17(10):1176–90.

59. Shen S, Jiang L, Xiao GQ, et al. Prophylaxis against hepatitis B virus recurrence after liver transplantation: a registry study. World J Gastroenterol 2015;21(2):584–92.

60. Perrillo R, Buti M, Durand F, et al. Entecavir and hepatitis B immune globulin in patients undergoing liver transplantation for chronic hepatitis B. Liver Transpl 2013;19(8):887–95.

61. Cholongitas E, Vasiliadis T, Antoniadis N, et al. Hepatitis B prophylaxis post liver transplantation with newer nucleos(t)ide analogues after hepatitis B immunoglobulin discontinuation. Transpl Infect Dis 2012;14(5):479–87.

62. Nath DS, Kalis A, Nelson S, et al. Hepatitis B prophylaxis post-liver transplant without maintenance hepatitis B immunoglobulin therapy. Clin Transplant 2006; 20(2):206–10.

63. Wong SN, Chu CJ, Wai CT, et al. Low risk of hepatitis B virus recurrence after withdrawal of long-term hepatitis B immunoglobulin in patients receiving maintenance nucleos(t)ide analogue therapy. Liver Transpl 2007;13(3):374–81.

64. Angus PW, Patterson SJ, Strasser SI, et al. A randomized study of adefovir dipivoxil in place of HBIG in combination with lamivudine as post-liver transplantation hepatitis B prophylaxis. Hepatology 2008;48(5):1460–6.

65. Gane EJ, Patterson S, Strasser SI, et al. Combination of lamivudine and adefovir without hepatitis B immune globulin is safe and effective prophylaxis against hepatitis B virus recurrence in hepatitis B surface antigen-positive liver transplant candidates. Liver Transpl 2013;19(3):268–74.

66. Choudhary NS, Saraf N, Saigal S, et al. Low-dose short-term hepatitis B immunoglobulin with high genetic barrier antivirals: the ideal post-transplant hepatitis B virus prophylaxis? Transpl Infect Dis 2015;17(3):329–33.

67. Teperman LW, Poordad F, Bzowej N, et al. Randomized trial of emtricitabine/tenofovir disoproxil fumarate after hepatitis B immunoglobulin withdrawal after liver transplantation. Liver Transpl 2013;19(6):594–601.

68. Stravitz RT, Shiffman ML, Kimmel M, et al. Substitution of tenofovir/emtricitabine for hepatitis B immune globulin prevents recurrence of hepatitis B after liver transplantation. Liver Int 2012;32(7):1138–45.

69. Tanaka T, Renner EL, Selzner N, et al. One year of hepatitis B immunoglobulin plus tenofovir therapy is safe and effective in preventing recurrent hepatitis B post-liver transplantation. Can J Gastroenterol Hepatol 2014;28(1):41–4.

70. Wesdorp DJ, Knoester M, Braat AE, et al. Nucleoside plus nucleotide analogs and cessation of hepatitis B immunoglobulin after liver transplantation in chronic hepatitis B is safe and effective. J Clin Virol 2013;58(1):67–73.

71. Khemichian S, Hsieh MJ, Zhang SR, et al. Nucleoside-nucleotide analog combination therapy is effective in preventing recurrent hepatitis B after liver transplantation. Dig Dis Sci 2015;60(9):2807–12.

72. Fernández I, Loinaz C, Hernández O, et al. Tenofovir/entecavir monotherapy after hepatitis B immunoglobulin withdrawal is safe and effective in the prevention of hepatitis B in liver transplant recipients. Transpl Infect Dis 2015;17(5):695–701.

73. Saab S, Desai S, Tsaoi D, et al. Posttransplantation hepatitis B prophylaxis with combination oral nucleoside and nucleotide analog therapy. Am J Transplant 2011;11(3):511–7.

74. Neff GW, Kemmer N, Kaiser TE, et al. Combination therapy in liver transplant recipients with hepatitis B virus without hepatitis B immune globulin. Dig Dis Sci 2007;52(10):2497–500.

75. Weber NK, Forman LM, Trotter JF. HBIg discontinuation with maintenance oral anti-viral therapy and HBV vaccination in liver transplant recipients. Dig Dis Sci 2010;55(2):505–9.

76. McGonigal KH, Bajjoka IE, Abouljoud MS. Tenofovir-emtricitabine therapy for the prevention of hepatitis B recurrence in four patients after liver transplantation. Pharmacotherapy 2013;33(9):e170–6.

77. Singer GA, Zielsdorf S, Fleetwood VA, et al. Limited hepatitis B immunoglobulin with potent nucleos(t)ide analogue is a cost-effective prophylaxis against hepatitis B virus after liver transplantation. Transplant Proc 2015;47(2):478–84.

78. Akcam AT, Ulku A, Rencuzogullari A, et al. Antiviral combination therapy with low-dose hepatitis B immunoglobulin for the prevention of hepatitis B virus recurrence

in liver transplant recipients: a single-center experience. Transplant Proc 2015; 47(5):1445–9.

79. Genzini T, Dos Santos RG, Pedrosa C, et al. Liver transplantation in bearers of hepatitis B associated or not with delta hepatitis in the age of the new antiviral drugs: is hyperimmune globulin still necessary? Transplant Proc 2010;42(2): 496–7.

80. Wadhawan M, Gupta S, Goyal N, et al. Living related liver transplantation for hepatitis B-related liver disease without hepatitis B immune globulin prophylaxis. Liver Transpl 2013;19(9):1030–5.

81. Fung J, Cheung C, Chan SC, et al. Entecavir monotherapy is effective in suppressing hepatitis B virus after liver transplantation. Gastroenterology 2011; 141(4):1212–9.

82. Ahn J, Cohen SM. Prevention of hepatitis B recurrence in liver transplant patients using oral antiviral therapy without long-term hepatitis B immunoglobulin. Hepat Mon 2011;11(8):638–45.

83. Sánchez-Fueyo A, Rimola A, Grande L, et al. Hepatitis B immunoglobulin discontinuation followed by hepatitis B virus vaccination: a new strategy in the prophylaxis of hepatitis B virus recurrence after liver transplantation. Hepatology 2000; 31(2):496–501.

84. Karasu Z, Ozacar T, Akarca U, et al. HBV vaccination in liver transplant recipients: not an effective strategy in the prophylaxis of HBV recurrence. J Viral Hepat 2005; 12(2):212–5.

85. Lo CM, Liu CL, Chan SC, et al. Failure of hepatitis B vaccination in patients receiving lamivudine prophylaxis after liver transplantation for chronic hepatitis B. J Hepatol 2005;43(2):283–7.

86. Rosenau J, Hooman N, Hadem J, et al. Failure of hepatitis B vaccination with conventional HBsAg vaccine in patients with continuous HBIG prophylaxis after liver transplantation. Liver Transpl 2007;13(3):367–73.

87. Yamashiki N, Sugawara Y, Tamura S, et al. Double-dose double-phase use of second generation hepatitis B virus vaccine in patients after living donor liver transplantation: not an effective measure in transplant recipients. Hepatol Res 2009;39(1):7–13.

88. Kim WR, Stock PG, Smith JM, et al. OPTN/SRTR 2011 annual data report: liver. Am J Transplant 2013;13(Suppl 1):73–102.

89. Kim WR, Lake JR, Smith JM, et al. Liver. Am J Transplant 2016;16(Suppl 2):69–98.

90. Cholongitas E, Papatheodoridis GV, Burroughs AK. Liver grafts from anti-hepatitis B core positive donors: a systematic review. J Hepatol 2010;52(2):272–9.

91. Joya-Vazquez PP, Dodson FS, Dvorchik I, et al. Impact of anti-hepatitis Bc-positive grafts on the outcome of liver transplantation for HBV-related cirrhosis. Transplantation 2002;73(10):1598–602.

92. Muñoz SJ. Use of hepatitis B core antibody-positive donors for liver transplantation. Liver Transpl 2002;8(10 Suppl 1):S82–7.

93. Chang MS, Olsen SK, Pichardo EM, et al. Prevention of de novo hepatitis B with adefovir dipivoxil in recipients of liver grafts from hepatitis B core antibody-positive donors. Liver Transpl 2012;18(7):834–8.

94. Saab S, Waterman B, Chi AC, et al. Comparison of different immunoprophylaxis regimens after liver transplantation with hepatitis B core antibody-positive donors: a systematic review. Liver Transpl 2010;16(3):300–7.

95. Lok AS, Zoulim F, Locarnini S, et al, Hepatitis B Virus Drug Resistance Working Group. Antiviral drug-resistant HBV: standardization of nomenclature and assays and recommendations for management. Hepatology 2007;46(1):254–65.

Toward Elimination of Hepatitis B Virus Using Novel Drugs, Approaches, and Combined Modalities

 CrossMark

Sebastien Boucle, PhD, Leda Bassit, PhD, Maryam Ehteshami, PhD,
Raymond F. Schinazi, PhD, DSc*

KEYWORDS

- HBV cure • siRNA • CRISPR/Cas9 • Anti-HBV agents • cccDNA • HBsAg
- Antiviral therapy

KEY POINTS

- Despite current treatments available for hepatitis B virus (HBV) infection, the inability of the host immune system to completely clear the virus can lead to incurable chronic infection.
- Identification of new targets and development of novel, curative drugs are necessary.
- New therapeutic strategies are critical components of a path toward a possible cure.
- A combination of antiviral agents targeting HBV replication, and drugs restoring or increasing the host immune response could lead to a functional cure.
- Novel modalities could disrupt HBV covalently closed circular DNA and also target integrated viral DNA.

INTRODUCTION

Over the past decades, research efforts have led to the development of several potent nucleoside analog inhibitors such as lamivudine (Epivir), adefovir dipivoxil (Hepsera), entecavir (Baraclude), telbivudine (Tyzeka), and tenofovir disoproxil fumarate (Viread), allowing a large decrease of HBV viremia in chronically infected persons.[1] Nucleoside analog inhibitors in their 5'-triphosphate form are potent inhibitors of DNA polymerase/ reverse transcriptase activities of the viral polymerase enzyme. They compete with natural nucleotides and act on several steps of viral DNA synthesis, including initial polymerization, protein priming, or the subsequent DNA strand elongation. It has been suggested that combination therapy using one of these nucleoside analogs

Funding source: This work was supported in part by funding from the NIH funded Emory Center for AIDS Research (P30-AI-050409).
Laboratory of Biochemical Pharmacology, Department of Pediatrics, Center for AIDS Research, Emory University School of Medicine, 1760 Haygood Drive, Atlanta, GA 30322, USA
* Corresponding author.
E-mail address: rschina@emory.edu

and interferon could have better virus elimination efficacy than nucleoside analog inhibitor monotherapy, but such studies are difficult to perform because the current monotherapy is already very effective at controlling HBV viral load. However, current nucleoside analog inhibitor treatments do not lead to HBV cure, as indicated by low levels of hepatitis B surface antigen (HBsAg) seroconversion (**Box 1**).[2,3]

Despite the success of current available therapy, subjects who cleared the virus (hepatitis B e antigen [HBeAg] negative, HBsAg negative) can experience reactivation of HBV on treatment interruption or after the use of antiinflammatory or immunosuppressant medications.[4] This strongly suggests that current anti-HBV therapeutics are unable to eradicate the virus from infected liver cells. These limitations have led researchers to continue their drug development efforts toward finding new viral targets that could potentially lead to the discovery of a functional or absolute cure (see **Box 1**).[5]

Considering that HBV covalently closed circular DNA (cccDNA) serves as the template for pregenomic RNA transcription, it is thought to be responsible for virus persistence. At the same time, integration of HBV DNA is thought to be associated with an increased risk of hepatocellular carcinoma development.[6] Accordingly, new therapeutic approaches that target cccDNA directly or indirectly are in development (**Fig. 1**). After recent successes with drug development for hepatitis C virus, the field of viral hepatitis is turning its focus to another major threat to liver health, namely HBV.[7] These new therapeutic strategies will have to address the problems of cccDNA elimination, intrahepatic innate immune response stimulation, HBV-specific immune response restoration and will probably have to include combination of drugs to target multiple steps of the HBV replication cycle.

Box 1
Definitions of cures

Apparent virologic cure

Sustained off-drug suppression of serum HBsAg, HBeAg, and viral DNA.

cccDNA = undetectable or repressed

Normalization of liver function (normal levels of serum ALT and AST).

Risk of death from liver disease: to be determined once long-term survival data have been obtained.

Functional cure

Sustained off-drug suppression of serum HBsAg, HBeAg, viral DNA, and cccDNA.

Normalization of liver function (normal levels of serum ALT and AST).

Comparable with individuals with naturally resolved infection.

Absolute cure – virologic cure

Sustained off-drug suppression of serum HBsAg, HBeAg, and viral DNA.

Normalization of liver function (normal levels of serum ALT and AST).

Elimination of cccDNA.

Presence of HBsAb.

Comparable with uninfected individuals.

Abbreviations: ALT, alanine aminotransferase; AST, aspartate aminotransferase; cccDNA, covalently closed circular DNA; HBeAg, hepatitis B e antigen; HBsAg, hepatitis B surface antigen.

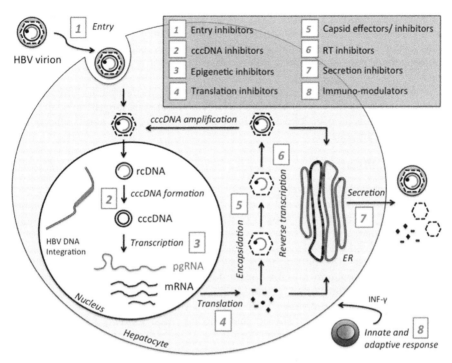

Fig. 1. Schematic representation of the inhibitors of Hepatitis B virus replication cycle. cccDNA, covalently closed circular DNA; ER, endoplasmic reticulum; HBV, hepatitis B virus; INF, interferon; mRNA, messenger RNA; pgRNA, pregenomic RNA; rcDNA, relaxed circular DNA; RT, reverse transcriptase.

New antiviral agents currently in the pipeline include entry inhibitors, relaxed circular (rc)DNA–cccDNA conversion inhibitors and capsid assembly effectors (see **Fig. 1**). Besides these direct acting agents, there has also been a significant development in the area of host-targeting agents. Examples include small interfering RNA (siRNA)–based strategies, RNA interference silencers, CRISPR/Cas9 approaches, HBsAg inhibitors, immunomodulators, therapeutic vaccines and Toll-like receptor (TLR) agonists.[8,9] Using these new investigational approaches, it is hoped that a functional cure for chronic HBV is achieved within the next decade. This review highlights recent progress in developing novel anti-HBV drugs and their mechanisms of action.

CURRENT TREATMENTS AND LIMITATIONS FOR A CURE

Nucleoside analogs are relatively potent inhibitors used for the treatment of chronic hepatitis B. These HBV reverse transcriptase inhibitors are usually well-tolerated and have excellent bioavailability. They are also cost effective in comparison to interferon treatments such as pegylated interferon alfa-2a (Pegasys) and interferon alfa-2b (Intron A). Nevertheless, these drugs have some limitations in terms of HBsAg clearance and cccDNA suppression. Although drug resistance can occur clinically with some of the earlier oral treatment such as lamivudine, drug-resistant viruses are rarely selected with the more recent drugs such as entecavir and tenofovir disoproxil fumarate. It has been thought that combination of nucleoside analog inhibitors could have an additive and synergistic antiviral effect and could reduce the rate of drug resistance. However, combination studies involving 2 nucleoside analogs did not increase virologic response, because the drugs are already very potent on their own.[10] As a result, because pegylated interferon has a different mechanism of action than a nucleoside analog inhibitor, their combination (tenofovir disoproxil fumarate + pegylated interferon for 48 weeks) showed a greater viral suppression and higher rates of HBsAg loss.[11,12]

As new therapeutic strategies are being developed for the treatment of chronic hepatitis B, uncovering new inhibitory mechanisms and potential targets, it is very likely that nucleoside analog inhibitors will have their place in future combinations with future drug candidates.

VIRAL ENTRY INHIBITORS

The HBV viral replication cycle consists of a complex multistep mechanism (see **Fig. 1**), starting with the virus entering the hepatocyte, followed by DNA replication, nucleocapsid formation, and release of virions. HBV entry represents an essential step for spreading and maintaining virus replication. The process involves 2 major interactions between the viral envelope protein pre-S1 and hepatocyte cellular receptors including first, HBV binding to the glycoproteins heparin sulfate proteoglycans followed by its interaction with the sodium taurocholate cotransporting polypeptide. Recently, Hepatera developed a synthetic lipopeptide, called myrcludex-B, which is derived from the HBV L-protein.[13] Studies have shown that the peptide competes with the viral pre-S1 motif for sodium taurocholate cotransporting polypeptide binding, blocking de novo HBV infection. Because of its early effect on the HBV replication cycle, according to the authors, the drug may also efficiently block the amplification of the HBV cccDNA. With this new concept, this inhibitor, which is currently in phase II clinical trials, could have a role in the development of an HBV cure regimen (**Table 1**).[14] Although, there are several other HBV entry inhibitors that can block the in vitro interaction of HBV with sodium taurocholate cotransporting polypeptide such as cyclosporine, ritonavir, ezetimibe, vanitaracin A, and irbesartan, among others; these inhibitors alone cannot lead to a complete inhibition of cccDNA synthesis as observed with Myrcludex-B. However, they might still play an important role by preventing viral entry into cccDNA-free hepatocytes when combined with other antiviral therapies.[15]

THERAPIES TARGETING COVALENTLY CLOSED CIRCULAR DNA
Covalently Closed Circular DNA Formation Inhibitor

HBV has evolved a unique replication cycle that results in the production of large viral loads during active replication without actually killing the infected cell directly. Two of the key events in the viral replication cycle of HBV involve, first, the generation of cccDNA transcriptional template, either from input genomic DNA or newly replicated capsid-associated DNA and, second, reverse transcription of the viral pregenomic RNA to form progeny HBV DNA genomes.[16,17] The HBV cccDNA is associated with viral persistence in HBV-infected hepatocytes.[18,19] Hepatocytes have a long half-life (>6 months or even years); therefore, elimination of cccDNA by hepatocyte turnover is not a major means of clearance. The major limitation of current treatment is the failure to eliminate the preexisting cccDNA pool and/or prevent cccDNA formation from trace levels of wild-type or drug-resistant virus.[20] As a consequence, HBV commonly rebounds after cessation of treatment with nucleoside analog inhibitor, leading different groups to develop assays to screen libraries of compounds to discover new antiviral candidates that can inhibit cccDNA formation.[20] In doing so, disubstituted sulfonamides, such as CCC-0975 and CCC-0346 have been identified as

Table 1
Therapeutics in development for the treatment of hepatitis B chronic infection

Drug	Preclinical	Phase I	Phase II	Phase III	FDA Approved	Target/Type
Nonnucleoside antivirals: interfere with proteins involved in virus replication						
Myrcludex B	———————→					Entry inhibitor
ARC-520	———————————→					RNAi gene silencer
ARB-1467	———————→					RNAi gene silencer
ALN-HBV	→→					RNAi gene silencer
Hepbarna	→→					RNAi gene silencer
SB 9200 HBV	———————→					RIG 1 and NOD 2 agonist
Rep 2139-Ca	———————→					HBsAg release inhibitor
NVR 3-778	———————→					Capsid inhibitor
Morphothiadine mesilate (GLS4)	———————→					Capsid inhibitor
AIC 649 (Bay 41–4109)		→→				Capsid inhibitor

(continued on next page)

Table 1
(continued)

Drug	Preclinical	Phase I	Phase II	Phase III	FDA Approved	Target/Type
CpAMS	→→					HBV core protein
EYP001	→→→→→					FXR agonist
IONIS-HBVRx (ISIS-HBVRx)	→→→→→→→→→					Antisense drug
IONIS-HBV-LRx (ISIS-GSK6-LRx)	→→→→→					Antisense drug
CPI-431-32	→→					Cyclophilin inhibitor
ARB-1740	→→					Cyclophilin inhibitor
Noninterferon immune enhancers: boost T-cell infection-fighting immune cells and natural interferon production						
RG7795 (formerly ANA773)	→→→→→→→→→					TLR-7 agonist
GS-9620	→→→→→→→→→					TLR-7 agonist

ARB-1598 — TLR-9 agonist

ABX 203 — Therapeutic vaccine

GS-4774 — Therapeutic vaccine

INO-1800 — Therapeutic vaccine

NCT01641536 — Therapeutic vaccine

CYT107 (interleukin-7) — Immunomodulator

TG 1050 — Immunotherapeutic

Abbreviations: FDA, US Food and Drug Administration; HBsAg, hepatitis B surface antigen; HBV, hepatitis B virus; RNAi, RNA interference; TLR, Toll-like receptor. Updated information can be found on the Hepatitis B Foundation website (http://www.hepb.org/professionals/hbf_drug_watch.htm).

inhibitors of cccDNA production.[21] These molecules are believed to interfere with relaxed circular DNA conversion to cccDNA in HepDES19 cells, also inhibiting de novo cccDNA formation. Further development of these disubstituted sulfonamides in combination with other antivirals such as nucleoside analog inhibitors might lead to the elimination of HBV cccDNA.

Covalently Closed Circular DNA Targeted Endonuclease

New promising systems that specifically use sequence-specific endonucleases to cleave cccDNA and eradicate it from infected hepatocytes have been developed, including the programmable RNA-guided DNA endonucleases (CRISPR/Cas9), transcription activator-like effector nuclease, or zinc-finger nuclease. Promising studies in cell and mouse models with CRIPSR/Cas9 have shown that these systems have the potential to serve as effective tools for the depletion of the cccDNA pool in subjects infected with chronically HBV.[22-24]

CRIPSR/Cas9 specifically reduced total viral DNA levels by up to approximately 1000-fold and HBV cccDNA levels by up to approximately 10-fold, in addition, it also mutationally inactivated the majority of the residual viral DNA in the stably transfected HepAD38 system. Moreover, these Spy Cas9/sgRNA systems showed additive inhibition of HBV DNA accumulation when used in combination with known pharmacologic inhibitors of the HBV reverse transcriptase enzyme in the Hep2.2.15 cells, and in the infected HepaRG cells, reduced both viral production and up to 67% cccDNA formation.[23] In an HBV hydrodynamics-mouse model, the CRISPR/Cas9 system was capable of disrupting the intrahepatic HBV genome ($\sim$28%), with significant a reduction but not complete elimination of HBsAg.[24]

SMALL INTERFERING RNA APPROACH

Persistence of chronic HBV infection is markedly demonstrated by an absence of antiviral immune response against the virus. As a result, a continuous production of surface antigen (HBsAg) in the plasma of chronically infected individuals is observed.[25] Three forms of HBsAg are secreted from infected hepatocytes, comprising filaments and spherical particles, with or without virion. The empty, noninfectious particles are the most abundant in the plasma, and may play a role in preventing the immune system from building a specific immune response against HBV. One way to stop secretion of HBsAg from infected hepatocytes is to cease transcription of messenger RNA (mRNA) by using siRNA. These short sequences of nucleotides (siRNA) knock down expression of genes of interest by promoting gene silencing at the posttranscriptional level. Several siRNA-based regimens are currently being developed and evaluated. The promising ARC-520 from Arrowhead Pharmaceuticals is in phase II/III clinical studies (see **Table 1**). This new molecule is composed of 2 distinct siRNA sequences, which was designed to reduce all transcripts of HBV cccDNA and with wide genotype coverage of the HBV genome. To enhance delivery to hepatocytes, ARC-520 was conjugated with cholesterol and then coinjected with a hepatocyte-targeted membrane active peptide. In chimpanzees, ARC-520 treatment resulted in a remarkable 95% decrease in HBV DNA levels and as great as 90% inhibition of secreted HBeAg and HBsAg.[26,27] Similar results were demonstrated in HBeAg-positive patients, however, insignificant suppression of HBsAg was observed in HBeAg-negative chimpanzees or patients, supporting the hypothesis that HBsAg in this case was produced from integrated DNA, which is not targeted by ARC-520.

TKM-HBV/ARB-001467 developed by Arbutus Biopharma is another siRNA regimen in a phase II clinical trial (see **Table 1**), which is currently being evaluated for its safety and tolerability in HBeAg-negative or –positive subjects receiving nucleoside analog therapy. This molecule targets 3 conserved regions within the HBV genome and seems to clear HBsAg expression from both cccDNA and integrated HBV. Lipid nanoparticles are used to transport it to the hepatocytes, giving it more stability against nucleases.

The siRNA-based approaches for HBV are especially beneficial because HBV viral RNA transcripts have their sequences overlapped. This facilitates the synthesis of a single siRNA trigger that could degrade all viral transcripts simultaneously and prevent viral proteins secretion. However, there are 3 main drawbacks with regard to siRNA approach for HBV therapeutics. (i) Specific delivery to hepatocytes in vivo: because of their small size and highly negatively charged hydrophilic phosphate backbone, siRNA are rapidly filtrated by the kidney and are cleared from the blood stream before achieving their target. (ii) The siRNA that reach the cell membrane of hepatocytes can be trapped easily in the endosome and undergo degradation by nucleolytic enzymes. (iii) Undesirable off-target effects of siRNA and innate system stimulation are also a concern. Despite these obstacles, novel chemical modifications seem to minimize the chance of cross-reactivity with human mRNAs to occur. These approaches can also enhance efficient delivery of siRNA to the cytoplasm where they can react with RNA-induced silencing complex and prompt specific degradation of the HBV mRNAs.[27]

More recently, Benitec Biopharma developed BB-HB-331 based on a similar approach pertaining to DNA-directed RNA interfering strategy.[28] BB-HB-331 is a recombinant DNA construct, capable of continuously expressing short hairpin RNA that in turn can silence permanently the targeted viral mRNA expression with a single treatment. They revealed the results of an in vivo study conducted in humanized mouse PhoenixBio, showing a 98.5% elimination of circulating HBV (reduced serum HBV DNA by 1.83 logs), a 94.5% reduction of intracellular liver HBV DNA, and almost complete suppression of serum antigens HBeAg and HBsAg (92.6% and 97.6%, respectively), and reduction of HBV viral RNA and cccDNA levels.

CAPSID ASSEMBLY AND CORE PROTEIN EFFECTORS

The HBV nucleocapsid is well-recognized to have an important role in the viral replication cycle. It is believed to play an essential role in HBV genome packaging, reverse transcription, intracellular trafficking, and maintenance of chronic infection.[29] Several small molecules including heteroarylpyrimidines have been shown to target the capsid protein homodimers that rearrange to form the nucleocapsid. They have been identified to disrupt the capsid assembly, thus leading to inhibition of HBV replication both in vitro and in vivo.[30,31] BAY 41-4109 (AiCuris) was the first heteroarylpyrimidine to be developed and reached phase I, but because of toxicity, solubility, and other issues, it seems to have been abandoned.[8] Despite hepatotoxicity in rats at a high dosage,[32] it was shown to inhibit the virus replication in HBV transgenic mouse[33] and, more important, effectiveness against lamivudine– and adefovir dipivoxil–resistant viruses.[33,34] Based on these results, HEC Pharm developed more recently another heteroarylpyrimidine named morphothiadine mesilate GLS4, which entered a phase II clinical trial in China.[35] Early studies have demonstrated that this new heteroarylpyrimidine was more potent and significantly less toxic than analog BAY41-4109.[36] GLS4 was found to misdirect capsid assembly leading to the formation of aberrant capsids without primarily affecting core protein levels.[37] Because these molecules may also have an impact on cccDNA stability, it is suggested that they may contribute to discovery of an HBV cure.[38]

Another class of small molecules known as sulfamoylbenzamides has been identified to interfere with the capsid, and potently inhibit the formation of pregenomic RNA-containing capsids.[39] NVR 3-778 is a sulfamoylbenzamide compound having a pangenotypic antiviral activity, developed by Novira (later acquired by Johnson & Johnson) that recently reached human phase IIa producing significant virus loads reduction (a 1.7-log reduction of serum HBV DNA and 0.86 log for HBV RNA, at 600 mg twice a day for 41 days). NVR 3-778 has shown encouraging pharmacokinetic properties, and was well-tolerated in human volunteers.[40] It has also been shown to inhibit the production of HBV DNA and RNA particles, especially in combination with pegylated interferon. Because their mechanism of action is still not completely clear, this new class of small molecules represent a promising cohort of molecules with curative potential when combined with other small molecule inhibitors.

TOLL-LIKE RECEPTOR

TLR agonists have antiviral effects. TLR-7 agonist activates the innate immunity by stimulating plasmacytoid dendritic cells to produce interferon-alpha and other cytokines/chemokines and induce the activation of killer cells as well as cytotoxic lymphocytes. Therefore, this new approach with agonist-induced activation of TLR-7 can trigger both innate and adaptive immune responses and may represent a new strategy to treat chronic viral infections. GS-9620 (Gilead) is a small molecule with agonist activity. It binds to TLR-7, leading to subsequent activation of several transcription factors, including nuclear factor κB and interferon regulatory factors. GS-9620 has recently entered phase II clinical trials in combination with tenofovir versus tenofovir monotherapy.[41,42]

Other Therapeutics with Potential

Caspase activators, RIG 1 activators, cyclophilin inhibitors, RNase H inhibitors, and therapeutic vaccines are also being evaluated (see **Table 1**). Some of these strategies, such as therapeutic vaccines, seem very promising, but are still in development and will have to overcome any possible toxicity and problems related to immune-enhancing approaches variable in treated subjects.[9] An impressive reduction of HBsAg has been demonstrated with the novel nucleic acid polymer Rep 2139-Ca (Replicor) alone or in combination with pegylated interferon alpha 2a in subjects chronically infected with HBV or coinfected with hepatitis delta virus.[43] This compound is in a phase II clinical trial and has the ability to block the formation of surface antigen protein by inhibiting the interaction of apolipoproteins with these subviral particles.[44] Recently, a new in vitro approach was developed to facilitate the direct interaction of small molecules with the human HBV polymerase. With a large-scale production of this enzyme coupled with its structural and biophysical characterizations,[45] Voros and colleagues validated their new system using a small molecule—metal-dependent and -binding modulator of HBV polymerase, calcomine orange 2R—which inhibits not only the duck HBV polymerase, but also human HBV polymerase. It remains to be determined whether this drug would interact synergistically with nucleoside analog inhibitors that also target the viral polymerase.

Another approach targeting microRNA could also have a role toward an HBV cure. MicroRNA-122 (miR-122) is a noncoding RNA involved in liver development and hepatic function, which has also been found to play a role in the regulation of HBV replication. It has been shown that miR-122 plays a role in viral persistence; a decrease in miR-122 is correlated with enhancement of HBV replication through a cyclin G1-P53–dependent pathway. Based on these observations, Li and colleagues[46] found that all 4

HBV mRNAs were harboring an miR-122 complementary site, revealing a novel mechanism by which viral mRNAs mediate host miRNA activity, contributing to the regulation of liver cancer cell proliferation, invasion, and tumor growth. Moreover, recent studies have shown that transfection of miR-122 expression vector into HepG2.2.15 cells repressed the transcription and expression of the protein N-myc downstream-regulated gene 3 (NDRG3), contributing to HBV-related hepatocarcinogenesis.[47] Thus, given the broad interactions of miR-122 in HBV chronic infection and HBV-related hepatocarcinomas, this miRNA represents a target for the development of new anti-HBV therapies.

SUMMARY

Compared with the currently available therapies that decrease and suppress the HBV viral DNA levels to undetectable levels, the new investigational drugs and approaches described herein have the potential to decrease or eliminate cccDNA and/or HBsAg. It is believed that combinations of antiviral agents targeting HBV replication and drugs restoring or increasing the host immune response could lead to a functional and perhaps an absolute cure within a decade.[9] After the recent success of therapy for hepatitis C virus infection, the viral hepatitis community has turned its focus on the discovery of novel HBV-associated biomarkers and therapeutic targets. It is hoped that the recent surge in anti-HBV drug discovery efforts will lead to the development of novel therapeutic strategies that could represent a path to cure for the more than 300 million individuals who are suffering from chronic hepatitis B infection worldwide.

REFERENCES

1. Kang L, Pan J, Wu J, et al. Anti-HBV drugs: progress, unmet needs, and new hope. Viruses 2015;7(9):4960–77.
2. Wei W, Wu Q, Zhou J, et al. A better antiviral efficacy found in nucleos(t)ide analog (NA) combinations with interferon therapy than NA monotherapy for HBeAg positive chronic hepatitis B: a meta-analysis. Int J Environ Res Public Health 2015;12(8):10039–55.
3. Chang J, Guo F, Zhao X, et al. Therapeutic strategies for a functional cure of chronic hepatitis B virus infection. Acta Pharm Sin B 2014;4(4):248–57.
4. Wang YJ, Yang L, Zuo JP. Recent developments in antivirals against hepatitis B virus. Virus Res 2016;213:205–13.
5. Block TM, Gish R, Guo H, et al. Chronic hepatitis B: what should be the goal for new therapies? Antiviral Res 2013;98(1):27–34.
6. Hai H, Tamori A, Kawada N. Role of hepatitis B virus DNA integration in human hepatocarcinogenesis. World J Gastroenterol 2014;20(20):6236–43.
7. Lucifora J, Trepo C. Hepatitis: after HCV cure, HBV cure? Nat Rev Gastroenterol Hepatol 2015;12(7):376–8.
8. Block TM, Rawat S, Brosgart CL. Chronic hepatitis B: a wave of new therapies on the horizon. Antiviral Res 2015;121:69–81.
9. Zeisel MB, Lucifora J, Mason WS, et al. Towards an HBV cure: state-of-the-art and unresolved questions–report of the ANRS workshop on HBV cure. Gut 2015; 64(8):1314–26.
10. Sung JJY, Lai JY, Zeuzem S, et al. A randomised double-blind phase II study of lamivudine (LAM) compared to lamivudine plus adefovir dipivoxil (ADV) for treatment naïve patients with chronic hepatitis B (CHB): week 52 analysis. J Hepatol 2003;38(Suppl 2):25–6.

11. Perrillo RP. Current treatment of chronic hepatitis B: benefits and limitations. Semin Liver Dis 2005;25(S1):20–8.

12. Marcellin P, Ahn SH, Ma X, et al. Combination of tenofovir disoproxil fumarate and peginterferon alpha-2a increases loss of hepatitis B surface antigen in patients with chronic hepatitis B. Gastroenterology 2016;150(1):134–44.

13. Urban S, Schulze A, Schieck A, et al. 10 preclinical studies on Myrcludex B, a novel entry inhibitor for hepatitis B and hepatitis delta virus (HDV) infections. J Hepatol 2010;52(Supplement 1):S5.

14. Volz T, Allweiss L, Ben MM, et al. The entry inhibitor Myrcludex-B efficiently blocks intrahepatic virus spreading in humanized mice previously infected with hepatitis B virus. J Hepatol 2013;58(5):861–7.

15. Verrier ER, Colpitts CC, Sureau C, et al. Hepatitis B virus receptors and molecular drug targets. Hepatol Int 2016;10(4):567–73.

16. Locarnini S, Hatzakis A, Chen D-S, et al. Strategies to control hepatitis B: public policy, epidemiology, vaccine and drugs. J Hepatol 2015;62:S76–86.

17. Schadler S, Hildt E. HBV life cycle: entry and morphogenesis. Viruses 2009;1(2): 185–209.

18. Block TM, Guo H, Guo JT. Molecular virology of hepatitis B virus for clinicians. Clin Liver Dis 2007;11(4):685–706.

19. Guo H, Jiang D, Zhou T, et al. Characterization of the intracellular deproteinized relaxed circular DNA of hepatitis B virus: an intermediate of covalently closed circular DNA formation. J Virol 2007;81(22):12472–84.

20. Zhou T, Guo H, Guo JT, et al. Hepatitis B virus e antigen production is dependent upon covalently closed circular (ccc) DNA in HepAD38 cell cultures and may serve as a cccDNA surrogate in antiviral screening assays. Antiviral Res 2006; 72(2):116–24.

21. Cai D, Mills C, Yu W, et al. Identification of disubstituted sulfonamide compounds as specific inhibitors of hepatitis B virus covalently closed circular DNA formation. Antimicrob Agents Chemother 2012;56(8):4277–88.

22. Kennedy EM, Bassit LC, Mueller H, et al. Suppression of hepatitis B virus DNA accumulation in chronically infected cells using a bacterial CRISPR/Cas RNA-guided DNA endonuclease. Virology 2015;476:196–205.

23. Weber ND, Stone D, Sedlak RH, et al. AAV-mediated delivery of zinc finger nucleases targeting hepatitis B virus inhibits active replication. PLoS One 2014;9(5): e97579.

24. Lin SR, Yang HC, Kuo YT, et al. The CRISPR/Cas9 system facilitates clearance of the intrahepatic HBV templates in vivo. Mol Ther Nucleic Acids 2014;3:e186.

25. Marcellin P, Castelnau C, Martinot-Peignoux M, et al. Natural history of hepatitis B. Minerva Gastroenterol Dietol 2005;51(1):63–75.

26. Gish RG, Yuen MF, Chan HL, et al. Synthetic RNAi triggers and their use in chronic hepatitis B therapies with curative intent. Antiviral Res 2015;121:97–108.

27. Sebestyén MG, Wong SC, Trubetskoy V, et al. Targeted in vivo delivery of siRNA and an endosome-releasing agent to hepatocytes. Methods Mol Biol 2015;1218: 163–86.

28. Mao T, Graham M, Kao SC, et al. BB-HB-331, a DNA-directed RNA interference agent (ddRNAi) for the treatment of subjects infected with hepatitis B virus (HBV), can effectively suppress HBV in a primary hepatocyte model [abstract]. Glob Antivir J 2015;11(Suppl 3):111.

29. Alaluf MB, Shlomai A. New therapies for chronic hepatitis B. Liver Int 2016;36(6): 775–82.

30. Bourne C, Lee S, Venkataiah B, et al. Small-molecule effectors of hepatitis B virus capsid assembly give insight into virus life cycle. J Virol 2008;82(20):10262–70.

31. Stray SJ, Zlotnick A. BAY 41-4109 has multiple effects on hepatitis B virus capsid assembly. J Mol Recognit 2006;19(6):542–8.

32. Shi C, Wu CQ, Cao AM, et al. NMR spectroscopy-based metabonomic approach to the analysis of Bay41-4109, a novel anti-HBV compound, induced hepatotoxicity in rats. Toxicol Lett 2007;173:161–7.

33. Weber O, Schlemmer KH, Hartmann E, et al. Inhibition of human hepatitis B virus (HBV) by a novel non-nucleosidic compound in a transgenic mouse model. Antiviral Res 2002;54:69–78.

34. Billioud G, Pichoud C, Puerstinger G, et al. The main hepatitis B virus (HBV) mutants resistant to nucleoside analogs are susceptible in vitro to non-nucleoside inhibitors of HBV replication. Antiviral Res 2011;92:271–6.

35. Manzoor S, Saalim M, Imran M, et al. Hepatitis B virus therapy: what's the future holding for us? World J Gastroenterol 2015;21(44):12558–75.

36. Wu G, Liu B, Zhang Y, et al. Preclinical characterization of GLS4, an inhibitor of hepatitis B virus core particle assembly. Antimicrob Agents Chemother 2013; 57(11):5344–54.

37. Wang XY, Wei ZM, Wu GY, et al. In vitro inhibition of HBV replication by a novel compound, GLS4, and its efficacy against adefovir-dipivoxil-resistant HBV mutations. Antivir Ther 2012;17(5):793–803.

38. Belloni L, Li L, Palumbo GA, et al. HAPs hepatitis B virus (HBV) capsid inhibitors block core protein interaction with the viral minichromosome and host cell genes and affect cccDNA transcription and stability. Hepatology 2013;58(Suppl 1):138.

39. Lam A, Ren S, Vogel R, et al. Inhibition of hepatitis B virus replication by the HBV core inhibitor NVR 3-778. AASLD Liver Meeting 2015. San Francisco, November 13–17, 2015. Abstract 33.

40. Gane EJ, Schwabe C, Walker K, et al. Phase 1a safety and pharmacokinetics of NVR 3-778, a potential first-in-class HBV core inhibitor. Hepatology 2014; 60(Suppl 1):LB19.

41. Gane EJ, Lim YS, Gordon SC, et al. The oral Toll-like receptor-7 agonist GS-9620 in patients with chronic hepatitis B virus infection. J Hepatol 2015;63(2):320–8.

42. Rebbapragada I, Birkus G, Perry J, et al. Molecular determinants of GS-9620-dependent TLR7 activation. PLoS One 2016;11(1):e0146835.

43. Al-Mahtab M, Bazinet M, Vaillant A. Effects of nucleic acid polymer therapy alone or in combination with immunotherapy on the establishment of SVR in patients with chronic HBV infection. J Clin Virol 2015;69:228.

44. REP 2139-Ca/Pegasys™ combination therapy in hepatitis B/hepatitis D co-infection. U.S. National Institutes of Health ClinicalTrials.gov; 2015. Available at: clinicaltrials.gov/ct2/show/NCT02233075. Accessed April 5, 2016.

45. Vörös J, Urbanek A, Rautureau GJP, et al. Large-scale production and structural and biophysical characterizations of the human hepatitis B virus polymerase. J Virol 2014;88(5):2584–99.

46. Li C, Wang Y, Wang S, et al. Hepatitis B virus mRNA-mediated miR-122 inhibition upregulates PTTG1-binding protein, which promotes hepatocellular carcinoma tumor growth and cell invasion. J Virol 2013;87(4):2193–205.

47. Fan CG, Wang CM, Tian C, et al. miR-122 inhibits viral replication and cell proliferation in hepatitis B virus-related hepatocellular carcinoma and targets NDRG3. Oncol Rep 2011;26(5):1281–6.

UNITED STATES POSTAL SERVICE ® Statement of Ownership, Management, and Circulation (All Periodicals Publications Except Requester Publications)

1. Publication Title	2. Publication Number	3. Filing Date
CLINICS IN LIVER DISEASE	016 – 754	9/18/2016

4. Issue Frequency	5. Number of Issues Published Annually	6. Annual Subscription Price
FEB, MAY, AUG, NOV	4	$282.00

7. Complete Mailing Address of Known Office of Publication (Not printer) (Street, city, county, state, and ZIP+4®)

ELSEVIER INC.
360 PARK AVENUE SOUTH
NEW YORK, NY 10010-1710

Contact Person: STEPHEN R. BUSHING
Telephone (Include area code): 215-239-3688

8. Complete Mailing Address of Headquarters or General Business Office of Publisher (Not printer)

ELSEVIER INC.
360 PARK AVENUE SOUTH
NEW YORK, NY 10010-1710

9. Full Names and Complete Mailing Addresses of Publisher, Editor, and Managing Editor (Do not leave blank)

Publisher (Name and complete mailing address)

LINDA BELFUS, ELSEVIER INC.
1600 JOHN F KENNEDY BLVD. SUITE 1800
PHILADELPHIA, PA 19103-2899

Editor (Name and complete mailing address)

KERRY HOLLAND, ELSEVIER INC.
1600 JOHN F KENNEDY BLVD. SUITE 1800
PHILADELPHIA, PA 19103-2899

Managing Editor (Name and complete mailing address)

ADRIANNE BRIGIDO, ELSEVIER INC.
1600 JOHN F KENNEDY BLVD. SUITE 1800
PHILADELPHIA, PA 19103-2899

10. Owner (Do not leave blank. If the publication is owned by a corporation, give the name and address of the corporation immediately followed by the names and addresses of all stockholders owning or holding 1 percent or more of the total amount of stock. If not owned by a corporation, give the names and addresses of the individual owners. If owned by a partnership or other unincorporated firm, give its name and address as well as those of each individual owner. If the publication is published by a nonprofit organization, give its name and address.)

Full Name	Complete Mailing Address
WHOLLY OWNED SUBSIDIARY OF REED/ELSEVIER, US HOLDINGS	1600 JOHN F KENNEDY BLVD. SUITE 1800 PHILADELPHIA, PA 19103-2899

11. Known Bondholders, Mortgagees, and Other Security Holders Owning or Holding 1 Percent or More of Total Amount of Bonds, Mortgages, or Other Securities. If none, check box → ☐ None

Full Name	Complete Mailing Address
N/A	

12. Tax Status (For completion by nonprofit organizations authorized to mail at nonprofit rates) (Check one)
The purpose, function, and nonprofit status of this organization and the exempt status for federal income tax purposes:
☐ Has Not Changed During Preceding 12 Months
☐ Has Changed During Preceding 12 Months (Publisher must submit explanation of change with this statement)

13. Publication Title	14. Issue Date for Circulation Data Below
CLINICS IN LIVER DISEASE	AUGUST 2016

15. Extent and Nature of Circulation			Average No. Copies Each Issue During Preceding 12 Months	No. Copies of Single Issue Published Nearest to Filing Date
a. Total Number of Copies (Net press run)			284	358
b. Paid Circulation (By Mail and Outside the Mail)	(1)	Mailed Outside-County Paid Subscriptions Stated on PS Form 3541 (Include paid distribution above nominal rate, advertiser's proof copies, and exchange copies)	65	81
	(2)	Mailed In-County Paid Subscriptions Stated on PS Form 3541 (Include paid distribution above nominal rate, advertiser's proof copies, and exchange copies)	0	0
	(3)	Paid Distribution Outside the Mails Including Sales Through Dealers and Carriers, Street Vendors, Counter Sales, and Other Paid Distribution Outside USPS®	52	63
	(4)	Paid Distribution by Other Classes of Mail Through the USPS (e.g., First-Class Mail®)	0	0
c. Total Paid Distribution (Sum of 15b (1), (2), (3), and (4))			117	144
d. Free or Nominal Rate Distribution (By Mail and Outside the Mail)	(1)	Free or Nominal Rate Outside-County Copies included on PS Form 3541	64	89
	(2)	Free or Nominal Rate In-County Copies included on PS Form 3541	0	0
	(3)	Free or Nominal Rate Copies Mailed at Other Classes Through the USPS (e.g., First-Class Mail)	0	0
	(4)	Free or Nominal Rate Distribution Outside the Mail (Carriers or other means)	0	0
e. Total Free or Nominal Rate Distribution (Sum of 15d (1), (2), (3) and (4))			64	89
f. Total Distribution (Sum of 15c and 15e)			181	233
g. Copies not Distributed (See Instructions to Publishers #4 (page #3))			103	125
h. Total (Sum of 15f and g)			284	358
i. Percent Paid (15c divided by 15f times 100)			65%	62%

* If you are claiming electronic copies, go to line 16 on page 3. If you are not claiming electronic copies, skip to line 17 on page 3.

16. Electronic Copy Circulation	Average No. Copies Each Issue During Preceding 12 Months	No. Copies of Single Issue Published Nearest to Filing Date
a. Paid Electronic Copies	0	0
b. Total Paid Print Copies (Line 15c) + Paid Electronic Copies (Line 16a)	117	144
c. Total Print Distribution (Line 15f) + Paid Electronic Copies (Line 16a)	181	233
d. Percent Paid (Both Print & Electronic Copies) (16b divided by 16c × 100)	65%	62%

☒ I certify that 50% of all my distributed copies (electronic and print) are paid above a nominal price.

17. Publication of Statement of Ownership
☒ If the publication is a general publication, publication of this statement is required. Will be printed in the NOVEMBER 2016 issue of this publication.   ☐ Publication not required.

18. Signature and Title of Editor, Publisher, Business Manager, or Owner

STEPHEN R. BUSHING - INVENTORY DISTRIBUTION CONTROL MANAGER   Date 9/18/2016

I certify that all information furnished on this form is true and complete. I understand that anyone who furnishes false or misleading information on this form or who omits material or information requested on the form may be subject to criminal sanctions (including fines and imprisonment) and/or civil sanctions (including civil penalties).

PS Form 3526, July 2014 (Page 3 of 4)   PRIVACY NOTICE: See our privacy policy on www.usps.com.

Moving?

Make sure your subscription moves with you!

To notify us of your new address, find your **Clinics Account Number** (located on your mailing label above your name), and contact customer service at:

Email: journalscustomerservice-usa@elsevier.com

800-654-2452 (subscribers in the U.S. & Canada)
314-447-8871 (subscribers outside of the U.S. & Canada)

Fax number: 314-447-8029

Elsevier Health Sciences Division
Subscription Customer Service
3251 Riverport Lane
Maryland Heights, MO 63043

*To ensure uninterrupted delivery of your subscription, please notify us at least 4 weeks in advance of move.

Printed and bound by CPI Group (UK) Ltd, Croydon, CR0 4YY

03/10/2024

01040397-0012